Alternative/ Complementary Therapies and Self-Help Techniques

A Guide
by Martin J. Hibbs

First Published 2018

Disclaimer

Please note*In the case of a specific health issue mentioned in this publication, before embarking on any of the therapies mentioned in this guide; it is very important to consult a doctor or professionally recognised healthcare professional, in order to get the very latest and most accurate information and treatment options available on any given health condition. Because of this fact, and having pointed this out, neither the author, publisher, nor the distributors of this book can accept any liability in respect to any bad outcome, following a "complementary or alternative" treatment, as mentioned in this publication.

Likewise; owing to the fact that guidelines and many "alternative" therapy methods of treatment employed (particularly in the case of aromatherapy oils for example) tend to change over time, as new research of effectiveness and possible risks of using or ingesting certain substances or undergoing certain procedures come to light, neither the author, publisher, nor the distributors of this book can therefore accept any liability in respect to any information deemed to be misleading or inaccurate within this publication. Being just a general outline guide to many therapies, it therefore remains the responsibility of any person reading this guide, and considering any particular form of therapy, to do more extensive and detailed research on any therapies they might feel inclined to try, before embarking on a particular treatment programme.

INTRODUCTION

This guide has been produced in order to help anyone who might be interested in, or might be wanting to know more about "alternative" therapies. This guide will also help those currently looking into some form of alternative treatment as a therapeutic option, to choose a form of "alternative" or "complementary" therapy which is right for them. In some cases, this guide will also provide information as to how people can help themselves and those around them to stay healthy, using techniques such as stress management, massage, and dietary measures. All of these later forms of self-help therapy will; if used as directed, help any readers of this guide to live a healthier life.

"Complementary" therapies are used quite widely these days; and for a very wide range of reasons. Whilst some of the therapies in this guide are covered in depth, the bulk of those mentioned are covered only in rough outline form to give readers an idea of the vast range of therapies open to them. Those wishing to know more about a particular therapy would be well advised to either contact their nearest practitioner, do some online research; or else visit their local library or bookshop where many excellent specialist publications can be found. Many such publications will have been produced by practicing authors in specific therapeutic disciplines of which they will have much in-depth knowledge.

This guide has been designed as an introduction to "alternative" medicine, and has been produced in two parts. Part one gives a basic outline to most "complementary" and "alternative" therapies, for the benefit of those who are new to, and considering "alternative" therapies as part of a treatment programme. Part two consists of a self-help section giving basic information on home treatments and ways in which we can help ourselves to stay healthy.

When assessing any of the "complementary" therapies mentioned in this book (no matter how implausible they may seem), it's important to realise that they have all achieved dramatically successful results in their own way. Whilst it is easy to be sceptical of things we don't thoroughly understand, it's also important to realize that for those who use such methods of treatment, these therapies often give hope and relief where most conventional therapies fail. Indeed hope and belief are without doubt, the mainstay of any therapy. If you believe you will be cured, you probably will be; if on the other hand you doubt a treatment will be effective then it's highly unlikely it will be.

Whilst some may be sceptical where such therapies are concerned, it has to be acknowledged by all that a great many therapies (i.e. aromatherapy, acupuncture, reflexology etc) are extremely relaxing. In respect to today's stressful world this makes them very valuable tools in the prevention of illness.

Complementary and alternative therapies (a definition)

Before going on I feel I should first explain the terms "complementary" and "alternative" medicine, although in actual fact these terms are self explanatory in themselves.

Complementary, dictionary definition, **meaning to complete, make whole.**

Alternative medicine, dictionary definition, **another option/choice.**

Complementary therapists for example, assist in providing a complete healthcare service to those in need, and give assistance to the orthodox medical regimes where necessary. Stress related illness and back and joint injuries being prime examples of the conditions which practitioners treat. Such conditions do of course require a considerable amount of time being spent, in order to help the patient reach optimum health (time which the average family doctor/medical practitioner can ill afford to spare, but which most "complementary" specialists have in abundance).

There are obviously many different therapies available which come into the "complementary" category (far too many for me to list in total), so I will merely summarise them here to give you a rough idea of the various therapies involved:

PHYSICAL THERAPISTS	PSYCOTHERAPISTS
Acupuncturists	Councillors
Aromatherapists	Hypnotherapists
Chiropodists	Psychotherapists/ Behavioural therapists
Chiropractors	Psychosexual therapists
Dieticians	Reiki therapists
Herbalists/Homeopaths	Spiritual healers
Iridologists	Stress consultants
Physio's	Visualisation therapists
Reflexologists	Yoga therapists
Shiatsu therapists	

As I've just indicated, the list is in effect quite endless however when you take into account the many variants which apply in respect to the many psychotherapists etc currently practising; practitioners who sometimes use the following mediums in a variety of ways to achieve their therapeutic aim.

1. Music therapy
2. Colour therapy
3. Drama therapy
4. Kirlian photography
5. Meditation

Unlike most drug treatments offered by orthodox practitioners (which target specific problems) most "complementary" therapists use a holistic approach in respect to their treatments, treatments which aim to seek out and treat any imbalances within the person as a whole. In effect they have 4 ways of doing so (depending upon their own particular therapy). Some will use predominantly physical means (masseurs, chiropractors, physiotherapists, chiropodists etc). Others will use counselling methods, (councillors, dieticians, psychotherapists, stress consultants, psychosexual therapists etc).

Others will use pressure therapies in either a physical or spiritual way (acupuncturists, reflexologists, shiatsu therapists, etc); whilst a fourth group will use predominantly spiritual/emotional means to influence our health (healers, reiki therapists, music and colour therapists, visualisation therapists, yoga practitioners). Many such therapists, use techniques which have been developed over centuries, to great effect; therapies which still work well in the modern age despite all the technological advances which have been made.

Medical science has of course moved on considerably in the last two hundred years or so, with greatly improved diagnostic and operating techniques now available. Drugs, x-rays, digital scanners and lasers are being used more and more these days. Despite these advances, there is still a great need for such specialist healthcare services; "Complementary" and "alternative" therapies certainly have a role to play in respect to our health maintenance and any corrective treatments that may be required. There are however a good many sceptics amongst the orthodox medical profession who question "alternative" methods of treatment, though in recent times even a large proportion of them are now having to acknowledge the need to have such therapists working alongside them. This being the case, "complementary" and "alternative" practitioners are sometimes called in to assist them with their most baffling cases, and deal with the many stress related ailments for which drugs provide no answer.

Another issue which can disturb the orthodox professionals, relates to the amount of food supplements and general cure-alls available at health-food outlets, and indeed non-specialist retailers (even mail order via the internet in some cases). Whilst such preparations are often perfectly safe in small amounts and may be beneficial, overdosing with these supplements, or using inappropriate aromatherapy oils can indeed cause conditions to become worse in some cases, and so many orthodox healthcare professionals are naturally very wary of such products. Indeed they are right to be, the unsupervised use of these products is indeed something to be worried about. It has now been discovered that certain natural plant extracts and food supplements widely available on the internet, and available through health-food outlets (besides being beneficial), may in rare cases, have a negative influence on the body too. In rare cases, some food supplements or plant extracts could stop certain essential medications from working properly if used in an unsupervised way. When buying such products from a health-food store, it is therefore essential to discuss your reasons for buying such products with the owner or manager of the shop so that they can advise you in respect to any medication conflicts that could occur. In these circumstances it is of course very important to tell the shop owner or store manager about any health problems you might have, or medications you might be taking. Sadly not all products carry warnings about overdose and medicinal conflict effects, or the need for supervision and monitoring in respect to these products. This particularly applies when buying mail order supplements and plant-extract products from the internet. Indeed I cannot emphasise strongly enough the importance of consulting a qualified practitioner or reading up thoroughly in respect to the choice of any such products you intend to use, before you start using them in a home environment. (Such research is also very wise in respect to physical therapies too of course.)

    As regards the term "alternative medicine," this in itself can cause problems with the medical profession - they often feel threatened or criticised by such language.

When the term "alternative" is used properly, it is meant as an alternative option to the man-made, chemical drug therapies; now widely administered by modern mainstream healthcare practitioners; the chance to use a more natural therapy. It's not an alternative to the practitioners themselves, but to the man-made drugs so often prescribed these days.

Another common misunderstanding which can arise, is that of medical status. Many people when coming to see an "alternative/complementary" therapist, regard them in the same way as their doctor. This is a mistake which needs to be put right at the earliest opportunity, so I make no apology for emphasising the point now.

Like other healthcare professionals, most "complementary therapists" have undertaken many hours of study and practical training in their various therapeutic skills. This does not however entitle them to assume the role of a doctor. "Complementary" practitioners are merely support staff and they expect their patients to maintain a good rapport with their doctor, and to keep them informed of the views and assessments their doctor has given them. It's not the job of your local reflexologist, aromatherapist etc to diagnose a particular condition; in most cases, they are not medically qualified to do so. They do however get clear indications as to a person's state of health when they are working on them. Where they feel there is cause for concern, "complementary/alternative" practitioners will generally direct patients back to their doctor for a more detailed examination or so that they can arrange for you to have more detailed tests at a hospital healthcare facility. In the main, most "complementary" practitioners concentrate on preventative measures, and respond to guidance from a patient's doctor rather than aim to replace them.

I am not for a minute suggesting that it is always necessary to get an orthodox medical practitioners' approval before undergoing any treatment from a "complementary" or "alternative" therapist, but I would suggest that in many cases of physical disorder, it is advisable to make full use of the vast array of diagnostic facilities which are available free of charge via the British healthcare service. Alternatively, where you have a personal healthcare insurance plan in place (particularly when you reside in countries outside the United Kingdom); it may also be wise to use that plan to get access to such diagnostic facilities, either for free, or at a reduced rate, before you visit a "complementary" practitioner for a full course of treatment.

It's also very important to know exactly where one stands in respect to the parameters set by any pre-existing condition, before embarking upon an "alternative" therapy, since some of those on offer may not be wholly suitable for your condition. Also any "complementary" therapists you consult, will need to know of any pre-existing conditions which may affect their ability to treat you successfully. Because of this, first consultations generally involve patients filling in a detailed questionnaire in respect to their health, or else their being questioned at length by the therapist who is going to treat them.

Like general practitioners "complementary" and "Alternative" therapists need to keep comprehensive records of their patients in order to chart their progress, and where necessary, make adjustments to their treatment programme, in accordance with any new developments in their condition.

Sadly there are occasions where individuals with health problems have excessive expectations in respect to what "alternative" practitioners can do and have become disillusioned with orthodox medicine. This being the case, patients are sometimes turned away for their own good, being referred back to their usual doctor for further consultation.

"Alternative" therapists will happily treat stress related ailments etc where their regular medical practitioner has no option other than drug related therapy for example, but it is quite a different matter when they are aware of certain disorders where surgery is still the best option. It would be wholly irresponsible to dismiss orthodox medicine in such cases, which is why I am making these points.

As with the orthodox medical establishment, a duty of care applies equally with "complementary" and "alternative" practitioners too. (This also involves the relaying of information in a form that patients can understand.) As well as wanting to ensure that patients get the treatment that is right for them; like mainstream practitioners. "complementary" and "alternative" practitioners are also keen to minimise the distress that a patient's particular condition is likely to cause them.

"Alternative" therapies are beneficial both in a preventative capacity, in respect to keeping people relaxed, and also in some cases, in helping to discover underlying conditions, of which the patient may be quite unaware.

In the case of reflexology for example, it is very common to find crystalline deposits in the metatarsal region (i.e. mid bones of the foot) which correspond to the heart and lungs. In most cases, therapists will keep such findings to themselves; since in all probability, they relate directly to the condition of the client's foot, and not the patient's heart. This being the case, most therapists are only too well aware that they could cause their patients unnecessary worry if they were to reveal such findings. If however the patient has a history of heart irregularities and they state during a consultation that they have felt off colour for some time, and suffer frequent bouts of indigestion, then in most cases, the therapist will refer them back to their doctor. They won't necessarily tell them what they have found, but instead will point to the patient's physical symptoms, and suggest that they had a check-up just to be on the safe side.

From the age of 18 a person is free to choose their own medical practitioner ("complementary" or orthodox) and a great many people do choose to use the services offered by "alternative/complementary" practitioners. In a good many cases, such individuals are only too happy to verify the benefits of such therapies, and are willing to give testimonies as to how a particular therapy has helped them (back problems being a prime example). There are many examples where orthodox medicine has failed someone and a form of "alternative" medicine has helped to relieve a certain medical problem.

As the pace of life increases, "alternative" and "complementary" therapies have an even more important role to play, either in respect to people needing training in relaxation techniques (i.e. in respect to yoga etc), or in respect to their needing physically calming treatments such as massage etcetera. "Complementary/alternative" therapists also provide a valuable service in supporting the many overworked medical doctors in the country too. It is also the case that unlike them, who have but a few minutes to see each patient, most "alternative/complementary" therapists as private practitioners, are able to spend far more time listening to, and advising each patient. This can of course be therapeutic in itself. This latter point is one which most medical doctors and other state registered healthcare professionals are only too well aware of, but sadly; due to the financial and time constraints put upon them, they are often unable to meet such needs themselves. Realising the patient's need for further care, they sometimes refer their patients to "alternative" practitioners, knowing that such therapists can spare their patient as much time as is necessary to resolve their particular problems, or can administer a calmative treatment which will benefit their patient greatly.

"Alternative" and "complementary" therapies are without doubt, the forefathers of modern medicine. Many of the methods and drugs used by today's medical establishment, mimic the techniques and plant extracts widely used in the past, but not always with the same degree of success. Where man-made chemical compounds/drugs are prescribed for stress related illness is a prime example of their limitation. It has now been found that in many cases, their effects are not curing the problem, but merely relieving a patients' symptoms. The drugs do very little to resolve any mental conflicts which may lie behind any mental or physical health disorders, other than to allow a reasonable period of sleep, or calm a patient down, so that hopefully they can resolve any conflicts they have, or change their behaviour, without any need for proper counselling. In some cases the drugs prescribed may become addictive, or they produce side effects causing more emotional distress too.

Whilst technological and pharmaceutical advances are to be applauded, it is important to realise that they are relatively new on the scene and therefore it will be quite a while before they can be wholly validated as therapeutic aids.

As well as the example of new drugs and their drawbacks, there are of course similarities in the field of physical medicine. For example, modern physiotherapy departments often use mechanical massagers of one type or another to save time and money. This sadly is another mistake which is being acknowledged, in that firstly, the therapist/patient relationship can suffer greatly by loss of physical contact. Secondly, in some very rare cases, damage could be done to the skeletal system by mechanical vibration on worn joints. Such things are far less likely to occur whilst similar treatments are being undertaken by "complementary" practitioners, since they tend to use natural non-mechanical methods to restore health in most cases. "Alternative" practitioners do therefore have a very important role to play in the scheme of things.

"Alternative" therapists also have many centuries of experience to draw upon when the need arises; something clearly of use to modern medicine, take chiropractic medicine for example, spinal manipulation has largely been the domain of chiropractors and osteopaths up until now. Fortunately, during recent years the situation has begun to change, with many mainstream healthcare establishments now starting to appreciate the wealth of detailed knowledge acquired by such therapists. In some cases doctors, consultants and administrators are even allowing "Alternative" therapists to work in hospitals, or doing training courses on the therapies themselves, and using "alternative" and "complementary" therapies to treat some of their patients. This can only be a good thing in that it gives patients a much wider range of treatment options.

PHYSICAL THERAPIES

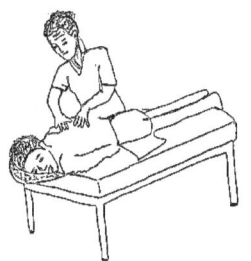

Massage therapy

Whilst many people are familiar with the relaxation benefits of massage, few people are aware of the therapeutic principles behind such therapy, and yet all of us at some time or other will have rubbed ourselves when we have banged an elbow or our knee. More often than not we have carried out these actions instinctively, as a direct response to some sort of pain and felt better as a result. This is a situation which has carried on all down through history.

Massage is without doubt one of the oldest therapies known to man. Whilst it is predominantly a soft tissue therapy it also has a great many emotional benefits too, making it a truly holistic therapy.

Sadly as a therapy massage has been greatly discredited by those in the sex industry, making many people associate it with a sexual service rather than a valid and extremely valuable form of therapy.

To understand this therapy properly it is necessary to understand a little of how our bodies work, particularly our muscles. As with most machinery our bodies require some sort of fuel. When we think of refuelling our bodies we tend to thing of materials we eat (many of which are broken down into glucose), they are only a part of the story however; besides what we eat, we are also nourished by the air we breathe. It is largely these two elements (i.e. oxygen and glucose) which combine to physically fuel our bodies.

Together they combust to give us movement energy, which fuels our muscles so that we are able to physically move.
As a by-product of this process, lactic acid is produced. In most cases our circulatory system will clear this via our second circulatory system (the lymphatic system). In some cases where our circulation is poor, or where we carry out very strenuous activity however, the lactic acid will remain and become crystallised. This is a situation particularly common in the neck and shoulders for example; where circulation is generally very poor (and also in the feet for the same reason).

These facts are the main basis behind massage therapy in that the masseur aims to locate pockets of lactic acid and any crystalline deposits and physically break them up, so that they may be dispersed and directed towards our excretory organs, and expelled from our body. As a result of detailed physiological studies it has been found that these pockets of lactic acid can in some cases bring about great disruption to our muscles, joints and neurological systems. This can often cause us a great deal of pain and discomfort (as many part time gardeners and hobby athletes will be only too happy to confirm).

In respect to the movements of massage - therapists generally work on specific sections of the body, working towards the heart. After they have carried out a series of long slow warming introductory strokes, they then work down through the tissue using their fingers and thumbs in circular motions to disperse any pockets of lactic acid or crystalline deposits (see self help section, pages 143-173).

The therapists working speed can make a considerable difference to the outcome of a treatment too (both in a physical respect; and an emotional one). Massage can be used to either stimulate, or sedate us, depending upon what we need at a given time; this being the case massage can be both relaxing, or in cases of depression, a stimulating experience.

Besides cleansing the body tissue, massage can also help us lose weight too. By working briskly, the therapist is able to break down fatty tissue and disperse it in the same way as with crystalline deposits. Though for such treatments to be wholly effective they should be accompanied by physical exercise and dietary adjustment as well (see also self-help dietary measures page 116 - 119).

As an added dimension to a massage, therapists sometimes use herbal plant extracts technically known as Aromatherapy (see herbal /floral therapies section, pages 32-38).

Physiotherapy/sports therapy

Physiotherapists and sports therapists, deal principally with movement injuries and rehabilitation following accidents or physical injuries caused through work or leisure activities; though in the case of physiotherapists, they also help with mobility issues generally, in respect to degenerative diseases such as arthritis, and age related conditions etc too. Whereas sports therapists tend to treat mainly short-term injuries, with a degree of fitness training and rehab incorporated in their therapy, physiotherapists will often be involved where permanent health situations apply and they generally come under the "Complementary" therapies category, in that most physiotherapists in the U.K. are usually allied to hospitals, state health clinics and other mainstream health care establishments. Such therapists tend to use a wide range of methods, including heat treatment, massage, re-tensioning techniques, or electronic equipment of some kind. Physiotherapy is standard procedure after certain surgical procedures, being a frequent tool of both orthodox and "Alternative" therapists alike.

    At a first meeting with a physiotherapist/sports therapist, a patient will be assessed in respect to their condition. They may be asked to show the therapist an area or a limb which is painful, or asked to perform certain tasks, such as raising their arm or leg as high as they can, whilst the therapist monitors their patient's level of achievement or difficulty.

    Once assessment has been completed, the therapist will decide upon a course of suitable treatment, or a supervised exercise routine of some kind.

    In some cases where direct therapy is required, therapists will often opt to use a mechanical device of some kind (often of the ultra-sound variety, see pain relief pages 87 - 88). In other cases the therapist will use a manual technique of physical manipulation (i.e. massage).

In most cases of physical treatment, the therapist will seek to warm the area affected before they start work. They may do this using massage movements - or where pain is great, or of a deep-seated nature, the therapist will use a heat lamp or a hot pad of some kind. Once the injured area of body tissue is sufficiently warmed, the therapist will then carry out any work they need to do on any affected joint or tissue.

From a patient's point of view, most treatments are carried out very sympathetically with very little pain involved in the short term, and great relief long term (provided you act on any advice they may give you). As a rule, their advice generally means resting the affected organ or tissue for a while, and then using the affected area with caution over a few weeks, days or months; whilst still undergoing regular treatments, until such time as the organ or tissue is wholly back to normal.

For some people however, physiotherapy can be a very time consuming, particularly so where a limb has been out of action for some time due to injury. In cases where a limb has been wholly inactive for a month or so physiotherapy treatments will involve gentle stretching exercises, repeated numerous times in succession, or else resistance work (where resistance will be set up against the limb to build up its strength). Both these processes can cause pain in some instances, especially so if the patient chooses to overdo any required exercises; this being the case, most therapists choose to supervise such exercise sessions and monitor their patient's progress very closely.

Chiropractic treatment

Chiropractic therapy was devised by an American (Dr David Daniel Palmer) in 1895 and centres around the working efficiency of the central nervous system. The bulk of treatments carried out involve spinal manipulation of one form or another.

Whilst chiropractic therapy is best known as a direct treatment for back disorders this therapy does in fact have the capacity to treat a great many other disorders as well. Probably the greatest merit of this therapy lies in the fact that many chiropractors insist upon working from x-ray photographs. This means that their patients can generally rely upon the correct diagnosis of their condition and suitable treatment afterwards, which may involve physical manipulation of some type.

Trapped nerves and slipped discs are typical examples where this therapy can be of great benefit. It is true that certain medication can reduce swelling, but no amount of medication can carry out manipulation treatments to correct misalignment of displaced joints or vertebrae.

In order to understand this most important of therapies, it's necessary to grasp the basics of neurological function; fortunately this is not as difficult as it sounds however. First and foremost, we have our brains, which via our senses of sight, sound, hearing and smell, direct us to physical action of one sort or another.

In order for our various organs to work they do need some sort of signal from the brain. These signals generally come in the form of electrical impulses which travel down from the base of the brain along the spinal chord/column, fanning out across the body to each of the relevant organs to be involved in any necessary action.

The spinal column is in effect a large wiring loom, like you would find in a telephone or traffic light sequencer box, with each nerve linked to the spinal column.

In all there are some 31 pairs of spinal nerves, plus 12 pairs of higher cranial nerves. It is these nerves which are the basis for chiropractic treatments; for chiropractors know that if any of those nerve pathways are disrupted, some degree of ill health or organ failure will result.
Workings downwards along the full length of the spine, each pair of nerves are responsible for various organs throughout the body. By feeling their way down the spine, or by viewing x-rays, chiropractors can tell where disruption is occurring. By careful manipulation, they can then realign any vertebrae/disks, or misaligned joints, thus restoring normal function to the tissue affected by such misalignments.

As I've already indicated, most patients visit a chiropractor when they are in great pain because of a slipped disk, or because unspecific back-pain of some sort. Because of their technique chiropractors are able via a process of deduction; to trace most ailments to some type of skeletal disorder. Once they have carried out any necessary realignments, they will then make some suggestions in order to prevent a reoccurrence of your problem.

As with most therapists, a first consultation will take much longer than any subsequent ones as the chiropractor will wish to conduct a lengthy interview as to how any injury has occurred and also find out about any medication being taken by a patient before commencing any treatment. In some cases a chiropractor may authorise x-rays to be taken before any treatment starts or seek access to any relevant x-rays that are already in existence relating to an area of injury.

In terms of physical treatment methods; chiropractors may use a wide range of techniques. Some chiropractors use purely physical means, to stretch and manipulate a patient's body by physically stretching joints, pushing down on them or pulling them apart so that they naturally realign. In other cases a chiropractor may use quick movements to twist and snap a misaligned joint back into its correct position. Other chiropractors will use specially designed manipulation tables to stretch and realign any areas that need adjustment. One thing common to both however, is the need to relax the tissue that is to be worked on before they do any work on affected areas. As with physiotherapists, this may involve a hot pad or heat lamp, or massaging of the area to be worked on before a chiropractor will start any treatment.

Chiropractors will usually recommend a course of treatment, say six to ten sessions, so as to ensure that any damaged joints are fully mended and working correctly. They will often give comprehensive training on how to avoid a re-occurrence of any injury too. Where a chiropractor suspects an injury to have resulted as a result of weakness in surrounding muscles, or in order to protect a damaged joint long-term, they will often issue a set of exercise routines to be carried out by the patent in their home environment or at work, so as to strengthen the muscles around any affected joint or joints. Once a chiropractor has seen you master these exercises in their clinic, they will then monitor your recovery progress over a period of several weeks, provided you attend a full course of treatment. In some cases a patient may feel better after an initial treatment and decide not to go back for further treatment. This may be because of financial constraints or because of serious time limitations but regardless of the reason, this can prove a big mistake, as upon feeling better, a patient may feel overconfident as to what they can do and suffer a relapse in their condition, which could prove far more costly in the long-term..

Osteopathy

Whilst it is easy to confuse osteopathy with chiropractic treatments, there are in fact fundamental differences between them in respect to their approach and the treatment regimes employed by each type of therapist. Chiropractic treatment for example is far more of a mechanical exercise, generally concentrating on an immediate problem, rather than the patient as whole. Chiropractic treatments are likely to last a relatively short time too in many cases; osteopathy on the other hand tends to be more of a holistic experience. Because of the in-depth nature of osteopathy consultation, treatment times are therefore likely to be much longer than would be the case with most chiropractic consultations. As part of their consultation procedure, osteopaths cover such issues as your general lifestyle, diet, and in some cases spiritual beliefs.

Osteopathy as a therapy was developed by Dr Andrew Taylor - Still in the 1870s and since the early nineties has been recognised by the medical establishment as a valid form of therapy, alongside its sister therapy chiropractic.

When undergoing treatment from an osteopath you will in most cases be assessed in respect to your muscle tone surrounding an area of sensitivity (i.e. a bad back for example). Following any realignment treatment (i.e. chiropractic type manoeuvres), or cleansing of tissue (i.e. massage therapy) that is necessary, you will then be advised in detail as to the various things you can do to speed up your recovery, or prevent reoccurrence of your condition, using postural, exercise, or dietary means.

Alexander therapy

This particular therapy is an offshoot of both chiropractic and osteopathy unlike them however this therapy centres round preventative therapy via our posture, rather than physical manipulation.

The therapy was developed by an Australian (Matthias Alexander) who studied both chiropractic and osteopathy in great detail from the point of prevention rather than cure. Being a very keen student of anatomy and physiology, Matthias Alexander looked for the solution to people's health problems and found that more often than not people's injuries and disabilities were brought about by incorrect posture over the long term. In his wisdom he realised that by re-educating people in respect to their general deportment, he could prevent a whole host of physical disorders.

The spine is in effect like a column of tiles with disks of cartilage sandwiched between each one, with neurological pathways threaded through each vertebrae. The straighter we keep this column of tiles, the more likely we are to keep them in place. If however we abuse our posture by the way we sit in chairs, walk, or lift things, those tiles I've just mentioned will become misaligned. This will cause causing wear to the cartilage sandwiched between them; and also, most importantly, eventual compression and distortion of our neurological system, which will quickly result in some form of illness.

Being only too well aware of these facts, Alexander therapists concentrate upon teaching people about more effective postural and deportment principles.

Rolfing therapy

Rolfing therapy is another therapy originating from osteo/chiropractic techniques. Like Alexander therapy, this therapy is predominantly concerned with posture and general carriage, though unlike Alexander therapy, Rolfing is very much an interventionist technique rather than an educational ideal.

The therapy itself was developed by Dr Ida Rolf during the 1940s and involves realignment of tissue, rather like Alexander therapy. In this case however, soft tissue is also worked on using very brisk, vigorous massage, and re-tensioning techniques, and so such therapy does not suit everyone. Rather than being regarded as a treatment in itself, this form of therapy is intended like Alexander therapy; to be preventative in nature.

Kinesiology

Kinesiology is in itself a fairly modern form of therapy having been pioneered during the 1930s by a chiropractor (Dr George Goodheart). In many ways this therapy is an offshoot of chiropractic therapy. Instead of relying upon spinal manipulation to treat patients however; this particular therapy centres upon muscle tone and overall tissue carriage (i.e. general posture at consultation).

As with other eastern pressure therapies, this therapy also involves the "meridians" principles, giving another dimension to the treatment in respect to supposed energy flows and subsequent blockages (see page 42).

Upon consultation with a therapist, you will be assessed in the same manner as you would with other physical therapists in respect to your posture and any pain or physical weaknesses you may have. In a good many cases, your diet will be taken into consideration, as will your general lifestyle.

As a therapy, this form of treatment appears to work very effectively in respect to neuro-skeletal conditions and can even have a positive influence in cases of allergic reaction as well.

Hydrotherapy

Hydrotherapy is used in a very wide range of contexts (including home treatments), and to treat a very wide range of ailments/conditions. This treatment is frequently used in a professional context where practical physiotherapy could be injurious to a patient's health, or where conventional physiotherapy would cause unnecessary pain. Water based therapies are known to be far less painful because they provide valuable support for those limbs or areas of the body which need to be exercised/worked on; this means patients can find it much easier to exercise.

Hydrotherapy treatments have many other benefits too. They can also work in a massaging context too (particularly where spa's/Jacuzzi's are concerned), in that during movement the water buffs gently against our body tissue, which improves our circulation. This in itself is known to be beneficial in helping to bring nutrients to our body tissue, and also in waste matter dispersal. In a good many cases, our domestic baths serve a similar purpose too. When we climb into a bath it can be for a very wide range of reasons other than to clean ourselves. We often use a warm bath to soothe our aching back for example. Not only does such bathing in a bath relax us physically, the hot water (or in some cases, cold water) has a physical effect upon our nerves and muscle structure too.

Chiropody

Chiropody is a well known and much needed form of therapy which deals specifically with foot disorders of all kinds, from foot infections, through to traumatic damage and deformities.
Chiropodists carry out a wide range of treatments, from massage through to beauty treatments depending upon their patient's needs. They will frequently recommend certain preparations to treat any infections we may have, or else some sort of device to improve the posture of our feet or toes, i.e. heel lifts, toe spacers etc.
As a therapy, chiropody is very closely allied to orthodox medicine, being used by both the disabled and the elderly for regular maintenance tasks of their feet.
Very often the elderly can have real problems reaching their toes to do regular maintenance tasks, and so for them chiropody is an essential service. Previously chiropody was widely available via the U.K. National Health Service, but these days, as a result of frequent cutbacks, the service is fast becoming a private practice only therapy.
Sadly the bulk of us tend to take our feet for granted and yet they are an essential part of our being if you think about it. Without them we are largely immobile (as many victims of injury will testify to). Whilst it is of course possible to get about by mechanical means, such methods are restrictive and inconvenient to say the least. This being the case, it is up to all of us to protect these precious resources as best we can.
Being foot specialists, chiropodists can therefore play a very important role in society, both in respect to helping us get over any foot problems we may have, and also; most importantly, in giving us long-term guidance in a preventative capacity as well. High heels are a typical example of this in that they are notoriously bad for the hip and back, as well as the ankles and foot, and yet most of us are unaware of these facts, it's only when we are in great pain that we discover this however. It is a sad fact but such

footwear can result in our being permanently crippled if we are not careful (something which most physiotherapists, osteopaths, chiropractors are only too well aware of). Indeed fashion has a great deal to answer for in respect to the health of our feet generally. It only takes a badly fitting pair of shoes for example and we can find ourselves in real trouble, this might be because of bunions, dropped arches, or arthritic toes, all are common conditions which chiropodists seek to treat on a regular basis, and yet they are all wholly preventable in most cases.

    In-growing toenails are another example where we are inclined to neglect our feet too. Sadly many people have found themselves in hospital where they have failed to maintain their feet and nails properly, or have worn bad footwear. In some extreme cases people's toes have become so deformed they have had to have them amputated. If we seek help for such conditions at an early stage, more often than not any problems we have can be put right, this seldom happens though. Sadly we are inclined to stick to bad footwear because it is fashionable to do so, and so such conditions often go untreated until it is too late. At the end of the day prevention is far better than any treatment of course and so it is up to us to get our feet professionally measured when we purchase our footwear, and wear sensible shoes rather than fashionable ones (i.e. flat shoes, rather than high heeled ones). If you do have problems with your feet, it is essential that you seek some kind of therapy as soon as possible. If you don't, you could have serious problems with regards to mobility in later life.

Colonic irrigation

As with many other therapies, this particular therapy has a very long history dating back as far as the Egyptians who believed that a large amount of toxins and harmful debris could build up in our digestive tracts, and be responsible for major illnesses. In more recent times the benefits of this therapy were brought into focus by a Russian scientist and biologist (Ilya Ilyich Mechnikov) who studied micro bacterial interactions and saw a link between certain organisms in our gut (living in stale food waste), and their ability to cause us harm.

As a therapy, this form of treatment is often frowned upon by a large proportion of society, both because of its implications, and also the physical discomfort it can cause. It is intended as a preventative treatment against cancer and other diseases.

Colonic irrigation therapy involves filling the colon (lower intestine/bowel) with warm water via the back passage and gently flushing the fluids back out along with any stale debris/toxins that have become stuck or trapped within our lower digestive system. Whilst apparently degrading and uncomfortable, some people (including many of high profile) remain convinced the apparent discomfort is a small price to pay in respect to potentially reducing the risk of horrendous diseases such as bowel/colon cancer.

HERBAL/FLOWER THERAPIES

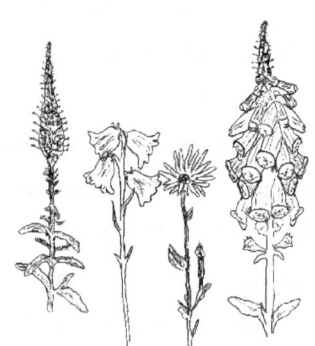

Homeopathy

As a therapy homeopathy is probably one of the most widely known of the "herbal/alternative" therapies being used today. Like so many other "alternative" therapies homeopathy has its roots in China and is still used as a main-stream therapy there (even today).

Homeopathy can treat a very wide range of conditions (both physical and emotional). After an extensive consultation period (which often includes an eye examination) the therapist will prescribe either one, or a series of herbal remedies. These will be issued for use in small doses, since it is known that many of the extracts used, whilst curative in small amounts, could do us harm if taken in too large a dose. Digitalis is a prime example of this, in that the plant is actually very poisonous, but in small doses plant extracts from this species can prove extremely beneficial in regulating our blood pressure.

Whilst there have been major worries in respect to herbal medicine and associated toxicity coming from the medical establishment at times, it should be noted that they do in fact use herbal remedies themselves in a very refined form. Digitalus (Foxglove) for example, is used to treat heart complaints, and taxol (a derivitive of the yew tree), is used to treat cancer these days.

Bach flower remedies

Bach flower remedies were developed by Dr Edward Bach in the late 1920s and are based upon the same principles of homeopathy (i.e. a minute amount of a plant extract taken internally will restore harmony to our bodies). With Bach remedies however; instead of the plant extracts being ingested in solid form they are taken in a liquid form, generally within a suspension of alcohol, being greatly diluted by the patient, who is required to add a few drops of the remedy to a glass of water. The resultant fluid should then be sipped slowly by the patient.

Unlike homeopathy (which aims to treat both physical and psychological disorders), Bach flower remedies are designed to work on our emotions, lifting our spirits and relaxing us. Probably the most widely used of these remedies being "rescue remedy" which is particularly effective at calming people down.

As a treatment, rescue remedy is especially beneficial when taking exams and driving tests, or where someone has suffered a shock of some kind (hence its name).

Aromatherapy

Aromatherapy involves the use of predominantly herbal oils and flower essences administered through the skin during a massage. Whilst there are many practising clinical aromatherapists, during recent times aromatherapy has become a very popular home treatment (see the home help section of this guide, pages 173-179), thanks to much publicity in women's magazines and newspaper features. Realising this, many therapists have set up teaching schools, and run regular workshops so that people can use essential oils in a home environment, which has also helped to develop this therapy into one of the most widely practised "alternative" therapies.

As a therapeutic medium, aromatherapy has a very long and distinguished pedigree. Like many other herbal therapies, aromatherapy has its roots in the Far and Middle Eastern countries.

By far the widest use of aromatic oils in ancient times however, were in Egypt and India, where they were used widely by the priests and holymen of the day, in the form of incense, and also by the pharaoh's physicians. Much evidence of this exists through the hieroglyphics of the pyramids, and also, through the scientific study of the pharaoh's remains themselves, as in the case of TUT-UNK-AMON. In those days, the oils used were of a particularly spicy nature; cinnamon, camphor and myrrh, being the most common. (Many of these, becoming available as a result of strong trading links with India, their country of origin.) They were at that time extracted from the bark of relevant trees.

In the Old Testament many oils such as frankincense and myrrh are mentioned as being precious, as later events confirm (when Jesus was born for example, where they were presented to him by the three Kings).

In the Grecian empire, famous physicians such as Hippocrates set great store by essential oils and carried out extensive tests as regards their therapeutic purposes, greatly widening their source to include flower petals, citrus and herb extracts. (Many of these being made available through the process of distillation, pioneered by the Greek apothecaries.) Hippocrates was also a great advocate of massage in itself as a therapeutic medium.

The Roman empire itself made use of flower essences for perfumes and skin tonics, many of which were extracted at great cost to beautify their leaders. In fact when such essences as rose, jasmine and neroli were being produced, the workers concerned with their production were stripped and searched every night, before they were allowed home.

From the middle ages, aromatic oils and herbal potions were very much the medicines of the day. In some cases those known to kill viruses and bacteria were used in sick rooms as a preventative measure against airborne viruses, to which the patients would have been susceptible.

Such essences as cinnamon, cloves and camphor have been, and still are, widely used by practitioners when appropriate. Even today, they can serve as an effective barrier against colds and flu type illnesses during the winter months, when so many germs are present in the air. Should someone have been unfortunate enough to catch one of these viruses going round during past centuries they were often told to gargle with sage or lavender. In the mid 19th century, yet more extensive tests were carried out, and it has been found that cloves of garlic for example, can wipe out tuberculosis, and, if used in the right proportions, thyme can banish typhoid and similar germs.

An interesting pointer to the potency of aromatherapy oils and their most recent history concerns a region in France, which was developed specifically for the production of aromatic herbs. A small town called Grasse, near the Cote-d'Azure was chosen as an early industrial base to grow herbs such as lavender, for products such as scented gloves (which were much favoured by the aristocracy of the time).
It was noted that whilst a cholera epidemic swept the land of their manufacture, the workers involved with the scented products miraculously escaped illness. Because of this, word soon spread in respect to the therapeutic qualities of lavender, and so lavender soon became favourable as a cure all.

Whilst the gloves idea went out of fashion, such items as lavender lockets and pomanders became fashionable, not only for their therapeutic purposes, but also as a basic perfume, to hide any unpleasant smells of the day. Because of the popularity of the herbs grown there, Grasse still remains one of the most important sources of aromatic oils, even today.

Towards the later part of the last century however, the use of therapeutic herbs and oils diminished greatly because of the advent of synthetic drugs, which were thought to be superior, and could be mass produced much cheaper. Their subsequent revival was largely brought about by a shortage of drugs during the First World War, when some physicians were forced to use more traditional forms of treatment. Because they were unable to get recognised synthetic drugs, many physicians started using certain natural oils to treat their patients, in an act of desperation. To their amazement, they found that the essential oils were in many ways, grossly superior to the drugs they had been trained to use, and found that the soldiers' healing processes seemed to be stimulated by certain herbs, oils and spices.

One particularly striking incident in the history of aromatherapy occurred when one of the main driving forces behind modern aromatherapy (a highly respected chemist by the name of professor Rene-Maurice Gattefosse), started experimenting with essential oils. On one occasion he was carrying out some tests on the properties of lavender and burned his hand very badly. In desperation to cool his burned hand, he put it into a vat of lavender. To his amazement, his wound appeared to be healing itself very quickly. Within a very short space of time, the burn had almost completely repaired itself. After this experience and the extensive tests which followed, the chemist concerned was able to verify the effectiveness of such oils, both through his personal experience, and also through his extensive tests.

You might be surprised to learn that there are a stock of over fifty recognised oils available for competent practitioners to use. With the help of these oils, it is fair to say that your local therapist can bring about positive effects in almost all cases, though there are a few conditions that they would not endeavour to treat. This is not because of the oil's limitation, but because of safety risks, as in the case of serious circulatory disorders, infectious diseases, cancers, or where surgery is required.

It would probably take me the rest of this guide if I were to give you a full run down of the people aromatherapists can help, but it's sufficient to say that all health problems (other than those I have just mentioned) respond well to aromatherapy treatments, in one way or another. As you will probably realise, it's much easier to mention those that aromatherapists cannot help, but just to give a rough idea of those conditions aromatherapists often treat, I will summarise them for you.

Stress conditions, insomnia, mild circulatory or skin conditions, P.M.T and P.M.S. symptoms, obesity, migraines and tension headaches, muscular aches and pains such as, fibrocitis and lumbago, sports injuries, the list is endless, but I hope these examples will give you some idea of their scope.

Aromatherapy is really four treatments in one, something which none of the other therapies can claim. Firstly, there is the aroma aspect of a treatment; aromas in themselves have the ability to influence our emotions, making us happy when we are depressed, relaxed when we are tense, thus helping us to sleep and being curative in stress related illnesses.

As I've already indicated aromatherapists can provide their patients with over fifty different scents, most of which can be used in the home, in the various ways I have already mentioned. The oil's aromas are in many ways just a by-product however. Their real therapeutic use stems from their constitution, and the vegetable hormones they contain. These hormones, can have great influence our own hormonal systems on occasion, and restore our health very effectively,) just like the plants they came from. We too are after all just a mass of cells and interacting chemicals, which are designed to work in harmony. This brings me on to the second, and probably most important point about aromatherapy, the fact that it is a type of massage, and does very much concern those cells and chemicals.

No matter whether it's the skeleton, skin, or flesh, all the body's organs consist of a complex group of cells, which rely upon neurological and chemical instructions to carry out their daily functions in one way or another (they also need a regular supply of nutrients of course). That's why we have a heart, to pump these various chemical messengers and nutrients around our bodies, to where we need them most.

The neurological system largely depends upon perceptions and experiences coming through the brain for its stimulation.

As I've already indicated, the neurological system is also closely interlinked with the body's glandular system, which works to bring about physical changes within our bodies (according to our circumstances). The hormones are carried, along with other nutrients, through the complex network of blood vessels, which run through our body tissue.

Without wishing to complicate things too much, it's important to realise that we also have a another major circulatory system called the lymphatic system, which deals firstly, with the processing of waste matter (dead body tissue, surplus fat etc), and also secondly, with disease, within the body itself. It's the lymphatic system which fights infection and repairs wounds.

Unlike the main circulatory system, which has the heart to pump it, this second circulatory system, relies solely upon muscle action, since the lymphatic vessels work through capillary action. During movement the vessels are squeezed together, making them pulsate, which pushes the fluids forward through the body's tissue. For this reason bodily movement is essential for good health.

As a result of this information, you will now appreciate just what a valuable therapy herbal massage is in respect to transporting the body's own nutrients and healing elements to where they are most needed, and also in stimulating the lymphatics to fight infection and carry out repairs where necessary.

With a basic understanding of the lymphatic system, you will hopefully see that besides being very relaxing; serving as a very effective therapeutic tool, massage can also aid slimming too, helping to remove cellulite, by breaking it down and moving it on to the various lymphatic glands, around the body. The same is true as regards morbid matter (which if the lymphatics are not working at full strength, can cause conditions such as fibrocitis, migraines and skin conditions). The lymph glands to which I refer, are, for those of you not aquatinted with their existence, situated evenly around our bodies. The main ones being found as follows, in the neck, under the arms, in the elbows, and behind the knee.

It has been known for many centuries that massage will relieve most superficial conditions and even some internal ones. It has been proven that massage stimulates the liver (the body's main nutrient store) and so promotes healthy tissue throughout the body. These benefits are of course greatly enhanced by the effects of the various herbs used in aromatherapy, and also by the various lymphatic drainage techniques carried out by a masseur, thus keeping our lymphatic vessels and glands clear of any blockages.

The third benefit of aromatherapy is of course the relaxation factor, that of all the nervous and physical tensions being soothed away, as the therapist works methodically over the whole body, kneading and cleansing the tissue, draining those all important lymph glands and channels.

Thoughts of these experiences are of course enough to bring about relaxation, something which many people find to be so, especially regular aromatherapy clients, who feel good all week. In times of stress they think forward to their next appointment, and so the risk to their ill health can be reduced simply by thinking about a forthcoming treatment session.

Aromatherapy treatments are also most beneficial in that they physically cover the whole body. They can prove far more beneficial in diagnostic terms than many other therapies too (though I use this term very loosely). During a course of treatment, the therapist gets used to a client's body and quickly notices if anything is amiss, through their skin colour, or in some cases, by physically feeling disorder within the tissue itself. In many cases a therapist will refer a patient to their doctor for relevant tests, thus reducing any permanent risks to their health. That is the fourth benefit of this type of therapy, in that it can act as an early warning system in respect to many serious diseases.

As a result of reading the previous pages of this chapter and having some understanding of our circulatory systems you will I hope appreciate why aromatherapists turn some clients away on occasion. As I indicated earlier, it is often in their best interest to do so. This is not because of the oil's limitations, but because of the risk to the person's health through over-stimulation of the circulatory vessels. This situation generally applies in the case of thrombosis, phlebitis, varicose veins, high blood pressure, and of course, where cancerous tumours are in evidence. With cancerous tissue, the cells could possibly be spread by over-stimulation of the circulatory system. This would obviously be detrimental to the patent, as would be the case with someone suffering flu type symptoms or serious infection, in that the spread of infectious bacteria or viruses could be increased.

With this latter group there is of course the other side of the coin in that the therapists could be at risk, or be putting their other patients at risk through treating contagious diseases directly (the most common diseases being serious foot infections). Aromatherapists do however have a wide range of oils which can be used to treat milder conditions such as athlete's foot and verucas indirectly. More often than not, therapists tend to issue oils in such cases, rather than touch the affected area themselves. Tea Tree and pachouli are probably the most common oils used to treat such conditions.

In some cases, therapists will make up aromatherapy blends, face creams and shampoos to help in a home use situation as well, though much will depend upon a clients' particular condition.

ORIENTAL PRESSURE THERAPIES

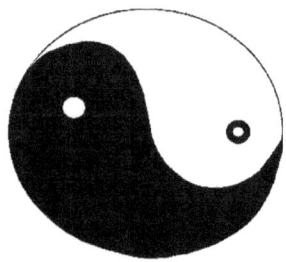

Oriental therapies work largely from a spiritual perspective with the philosophy that our life-force is governed by both positive and negative elements, which flow through the body in equal amounts, along designated body channels (or meridians as they are technically known). The main principle in these type of therapies, lies in harmony of both the positive and the negative (i.e. the yin and yang).

It is a widely held belief that should one of these elements become too dominant, then ill health will result; therefore when we are being treated by a therapist specialising in oriental medicines (i.e. a reflexologist, a shiatsu therapist, an acupressure therapist or an acupuncturist), they will be seeking to restore a sort of spiritual harmony to our bodies. Slowly and carefully they will work to unblock our energy channels. With the exception of acupuncture (where they use needles to restore harmony), the therapist will apply short bursts of pressure with their thumbs and fingertips as appropriate to our condition. Although such movements might at first sound uncomfortable, they are in fact very relaxing in most cases (including acupuncture).

Whilst it can be difficult to understand the Eastern philosophies in respect to chi (life-force) the meridians (energy channels) etc, there can be no doubt that these Eastern therapies can have a definite therapeutic effect/influence upon our central nervous system. This being the case they do most certainly have a role to play in Western medicine.

Acupuncture

Although acupuncture has been in use for many centuries in the east (and during the last few centuries in Europe), here in Great Britain, modern refined forms of this therapy have widely been available to us since the 1950s. Since that time, the therapy has become very popular and has achieved a tremendous record of success in treating a wide range of medical conditions.

The insertion of long needles into our bodies might sound very painful, but in actual fact the experience is quite painless, and in a great many cases, a wholly relaxing experience (as well as being physically effective). As I've already indicated, the essence of this therapy centres round our having supposedly blocked or disrupted energy channels. This being the case, the therapist inserts the needles into specific areas along spiritual energy channels called meridians, to restore harmony to our bodies, thus relieving us of the physical disorder which has afflicted us.

In most cases treatment seeks to relieve physical discomfort, but can and does work equally well on many mental conditions as well, i.e. insomnia, stress, depression etc. By far its greatest claim however, lies in the therapy's ability to relieve pain. Fortunately for this therapy, this particular trait has won it many converts in the mainstream medical profession, in that time and again the doctors have seen the most challenging conditions in their patients relieved after only a few sessions spent having referred them to such a therapist.

Shiatsu

Shiatsu and acupressure are very similar to acupuncture but without the needles. They are both carried out using the fingers and thumbs to sedate or stimulate certain nerves throughout the body. With shiatsu however, the patients are also given a wide range of manipulation and re-tensioning (i.e. stretching) treatment during the therapy sessions.

Shiatsu treatments are generally carried out on the floor, either in a person's home, or in a purpose built clinic with plenty of space. This is especially necessary with shiatsu since the therapist will in most cases require uncluttered access to their patient, and wish to stretch out the patient's legs and arms according to the areas they are working on.

Since each treatment is individual to the patient there is no set routine to speak of. After a lengthy consultation, the therapist is free to carry out treatment in whichever manner they choose according to a patient's symptoms.

One major advantage to this therapy is the fact that patients can remain fully clothed whilst undergoing treatment, though it is of course helpful to the therapist if the patient's clothing is loose in nature.

Acupressure

As a therapeutic tool, acupressure can prove particularly invaluable in cases of chronic or acute pain, particularly in home situations. It is frequently the case that pain is referred. That is to say if a vertebrae in the neck for example is displaced, it is quite common for the person to suffer pins and needles in his or her forearm, whereas the actual problem lies in the neck.

With training from a qualified shiatsu, or acupuncturist, or by using one of the many books available on this invaluable home therapy; it is possible to locate the origins of a painful condition. Simply by inserting your finger or thumb at certain points in the wrist, elbow, shoulder, neck, knee, hip or thigh, for a few seconds at a time; it is possible to relieve such things as headaches arthritic pains etc, in a wholly drug-free and non mechanical way. As with all painful conditions however; acupressure should only be used as an emergency measure, or where a definite diagnosis has been made by a qualified medical practitioner, or where extensive tests have been carried out in respect to a pre-existing condition.

Reflexology

Like most other pressure therapies (i.e. shiatsu, acupressure, etc), reflexology, works on the meridians, or energy lines, which run through the body. By working on these energy lines and zones, the therapist can actually influence the body's functions, (points which will be covered again in the following pages, since they provide the backbone of this important therapy).

Reflexology also serves as a very effective foot massage as well, by helping to clear the lower leg of harmful toxins, thus reducing the risk of serious foot disorders developing.

Please note - when referring to its use as a foot massage I am merely stating its most obvious therapeutic benefit not its limitation, so please do not underestimate reflexology's effectiveness as a treatment for the whole body. As you will later come to see; this is in fact a very effective treatment for the whole person. For a true understanding of Reflex Zone Therapy it is important to know a little about its history and how it developed alongside other "complementary" therapies.

Reflexology is often thought to have been developed by the Chinese along with the other "complementary" therapies. There's certainly no doubt that the Chinese are world leaders in acupuncture techniques, being largely responsible for their world-wide development and acclaim.

Anyone studying oriental therapies will soon see that there are many similarities between acupuncture and reflexology, so it is not unreasonable to assume that China has a part to play in the history and development of reflexology.

It is known for example that way back in 1017 AD an eminent Chinese therapist had a figure cast in bronze, with all the acupuncture points clearly marked on the feet. By using the figure for reference, the acupuncture therapist could apply pressure to the relevant areas of the patient's feet, as well as using the conventional needles to improve the energy flow around the patient's body.

There is much documentation relating to acupuncture in the Chinese archives, but very little available in the case of Reflex Zone Therapy itself, so it is almost certainly the case that reflexology gave way to acupuncture as the main therapy of China many centuries ago

By far the oldest documentation relating to reflexology, does in fact come not from China, as you would expect, but from Egypt and the Middle East. Pictographs have been found on the walls of various burial chambers belonging to the pharaohs.

Further evidence of foot massage in the Middle East comes of course from the scriptures. One of the greatest healer of all times, Jesus himself, used to work on people's feet, being only too well aware of their importance for good health. There is also evidence that the American Indians have for centuries acknowledged the importance of energy flows and general health in relation to the condition of their feet.

They as hunters were only too well aware that their lives depended upon the wellbeing of their feet and that their hunting skills were completely useless if they fell lame. The Indians believed that feet were sacred because of their contact with the ground, and so tribal healers concentrated upon them in a bid to balance their patient's energy flow.

Sadly reflexology lost its appeal with its original exponents and was apparently lost to medicine for quite some time. It was however; re-discovered by the Germans when they were studying the pressure and massage therapies during the latter part of the 1800s (having brought back into the public gaze, reflexology was then taken up by the Americans).

One particular therapist (a Dr Fitzgerald) did much medical research on the subject of reflex zones, and learned to influence the neurological system, by blocking various nerve paths with his fingers and thumbs. Dr Fitzgerald found that he was able to trace the energy or neurological zones very precisely, and effectively, thus verifying and guaranteeing the continued success and learning of this ancient therapy. Dr Fitzgerald drew up many charts relating to the body's energy zones, and split the body up into ten segments; thus modern Reflex Zone Therapy or Reflexology was born. Dr Fitzgerald's work was further developed by Eunice Ingham, who studied his charts and carried out her own exhaustive tests. She drew up a more detailed picture of the body's reflex zones and proved to be a highly successful practitioner in her own right.

Eventually Eunice Ingham went on to teach and write books on the subject, providing this unique and most valuable of therapies with the opportunity to grow and flourish as it does today (with at least one therapist in almost every town).

As with many other pressure therapies, there is much disagreement in respect the spiritual element of this ancient treatment. Therefore in this attempt to explain how the therapy works, I will purposely stick to the charts and facts laid down by Dr Fitzgerald and Eunice Ingham, which I mentioned earlier.

Dr Fitzgerald identified 10 reflex zones running through the body, which is how the term "Reflex Zone Therapy " came about. He split the body up into 10 vertical zones.

If you work out from the centre of the umbilical button, dividing each side into 5 sections, then mentally transfer them to the feet (5 on each side) you then have the basic zones. Zone 1 for example, runs from the nose down to the groin, taking in and incorporating the spine.

If you transfer this mentally to the feet, it corresponds with the medial aspect of both feet. If you examine their shape, you will see the skeletal shape does in fact match the spine, almost exactly. Likewise Zone 5 runs from the ears down the shoulders, arms and legs, when transferred to the feet. Therefore zone 5 covers both lateral aspects of the feet when they are placed together before you.

In the 1970's, a further 3 zones were identified and added. These last 3 zones came about by subdividing the body into 3 horizontal sections. For example, section 1, is the head and neck. Section 2, relates to the thorax, and section 3, the abdominal region.

These last three are perhaps the easiest for the layman to interpret. The first zone relating to the head and neck, is to be found spread across all 5 toes of both feet. The second zone, relating to the thorax, is to be found beneath the hard area of skin which covers the metatarsal regions of both feet. Lastly the third zone, relating to the abdominal region, lies immediately beneath the 5 metatarsals and runs down towards the ankle.

As I've just indicated, the feet are in effect a mirror image of the body itself; and as with normal massage, the therapists will work carefully and thoroughly on each zone with their thumbs in order to clear any crystalline deposits from the corresponding joints and muscles etc. They will also work very carefully up, down, and across the relevant lines, to unblock the energy paths, pausing on each gland and lymphatic point where necessary.

Should the therapist feel there is an imbalance in any organ, they will work specifically on the relevant zone until the patient's symptoms have eased. This may take one visit or it may take several, whichever is the case, there is generally some degree of relief to the patient. Great care is taken by each therapist to cover the whole of the foot, right up to the Achilles tendon, assessing each zone in turn as to its sensitivity, and the patient's reaction during therapy. If an organ is congested, granular deposits are often evident beneath the thumb as the therapist works.

In the case of inflammation, the relevant zone is tender to touch and needs to be worked on until the pain has eased. Usually the therapist will make an overall assessment of both feet before starting work on any sensitive zones.

The whole treatment usually lasts between 45 minutes to 1 hour, depending upon the amount of work that needs to be done upon the various zones.

As with most therapies, treatment procedures do vary from therapist to therapist, since each practitioner has their own way of doing things; but there are certain elements common to all. Firstly, having made contact with a practitioner and arrived at their door, you will be requested to fill out some sort of health questionnaire for the therapist's case history notes. You will then be invited to remove your footwear and climb up onto a couch, or sit in a special treatment chair of some kind, or if it is to be by way of a home visit; you will then be asked to make yourself comfortable in a favourite chair (usually with your feet elevated to the therapists' working height).

The therapist will then wrap your feet in a towel and ask you as to which medium you would like them to use. Generally the therapist will use some form of talcum powder, or you could be offered a blend of aromatherapy oils, which adds an extra dimension to the treatment (provided the practitioner is appropriately qualified to use them). Then again your practitioner may prefer to use just a plain vegetable oil medium.

Every therapist has their own set routine for working and the movements concerned so it would be wrong of me to quote a standard procedure. However I can point out that all therapists work with their thumbs all round the feet, covering up whichever foot is not being worked on at any one time.

For those who feel a bit squeamish at the thought of having your feet worked on, I can assure you that it is very pleasant and the movements used by each therapist are sufficient to overcome any ticklish sensations. For the most part therapists, are taught to note the various degrees of sensitivity and to work accordingly. In the past it was thought that therapy needed to be ultra firm, to the point of being painful; fortunately this view has long since expired.

The current thinking is that a treatment needs to be firm enough not to be ticklish, but not so firm that a patient feels constant discomfort. Should someone find a particular therapist causes them great discomfort then it's probably best to find another one. Please don't be rash enough to blame the therapy itself. As many thousands of people will confirm, it is generally a most relaxing and pleasant experience if carried out correctly, so much so in fact that the reflexology patients often drift off to sleep during treatment.

When most patients are asked how they feel after treatment, they frequently reply by saying that they feel like they're walking on air (a feeling which apparently lasts for several days). Presumably that is because all their muscles are relaxed and working in total harmony (a point which I shall cover in more detail shortly).

As with the other therapies in this guide, to fully appreciate this particular therapy it's important to acknowledge the essential role our circulatory system plays in respect to our well-being; by doing so you will be able to fully appreciate the following points. The first of which relates to the circulation of nutrients around the body (a task which the heart is largely responsible for).

Day in and day out our hearts pump nutrient filled blood round our bodies, taking nutrients such as oxygen etc to each of our body's cells. If you think about this, and where the heart is situated, you will soon realise that the feet are the furthest organs from the heart. To make things worse, we as humans walk upright, and so our circulation therefore faces an insurmountable challenge of having to work against gravity where our legs are concerned.

It is true that there are many valves in the leg to prevent backflow, but these do not always do their jobs as well as they might however. This being the case, our feet are very prone to poor circulation and are often starved of vital nutrients because of vascular congestion (odema and varicose veins being two prime examples of such disorder).

Whilst reflexology cannot cure such conditions, regular treatments and good foot-care generally, can go a long way to help identify and mitigate such conditions.

Our lymphatic system, which regulates our immune system and deals with waste products from the body's cells and organs, encounters similar problems too. This second circulatory system has no pump of its own and relies solely upon muscular action to function efficiently.

As I have already indicated, there is frequently a problem where the feet are concerned, because like the blood, our lymph fluids have to fight against gravity. Where inefficiency occurs, this can cause infected or waste matter to accumulate in the feet and their joints.

There are some 26 bones in the foot, all of which interact with one another to give us full mobility. If the joints between the bones, or the muscles which operate them become too congested, serious problems can arise. The most common being degenerative arthritis. Sadly most of us grossly undervalue our feet and it is only when we have such problems that we come to realise their importance.

Some people go through life without any problems with their feet at all; they however are unfortunately the minority. As most of us get older we do have problems. That is where reflexology comes into its own as a preventative therapy, by stimulating the circulatory system of the feet and in improving their condition.

For most people, a reflexology treatment every so often would do them a power of good. There are certain circumstances where reflexology is inadvisable however, where you have a history of serious circulatory disorders such as high blood pressure, phlebitis, or very bad varicose veins for example. (Any condition where stimulating the blood supply could prove harmful.) The same applies in the case of foot infections, foot injuries, cancerous tumours, or when suffering from flu type viruses too. Such restrictions do in fact apply to most "complementary" therapies. It is therefore advisable to consult your family doctor before committing yourself to reflex zone therapy in such cases.

Should your doctor advise against reflexology and you feel you need some kind of treatment on your feet, then it would probably be a good idea to ask your doctor for a list of reputable chiropodists who practice in your area. (See Pages 29-31 for details of the services they provide). If you are told it is O.K. to have a reflexology treatment, be sure to tell your therapist of any current conditions before they start to treat you.

Apart from these few exceptions relating to serious circulatory disorders, there really is no better therapy for the feet than Reflex Zone Therapy. It has so many advantages over other forms of treatment, too many to mention here, so I will merely summarise the therapy's many virtues for you now -

Firstly; this therapy can be very effective in respect to keeping the feet and indeed the whole body healthy.

Secondly; this therapy has great benefits in respect to its use for general relaxation purposes.

Thirdly (and I use this term very loosely); this therapy can have great benefit as a diagnostic medium.

Fourthly; this therapy has great convenience in that treatment can be carried out almost anywhere, without the clients needing to disrobe.

Finally; there is no risk of side effects from drugs.

SPIRITUAL THERAPIES

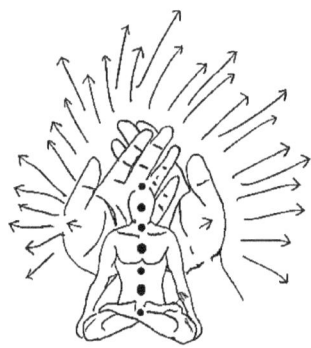

Spiritual healers

Whilst they are very difficult to verify and even harder to understand, spiritual healing therapies do indeed have a very important part to play in modern medicine. Not only do they offer people a drug free option in respect to their illness, most importantly, they are sometimes on rare occasions, successful in treating those conditions for which a cure is deemed unattainable.

Spiritual healing is a phenomena which has gone on all through history. Probably the most widely known healer in the Western world being Jesus of Nazareth, who brought much publicity to this most miraculous of therapies. It is a therapy where the apparently incurable have seemingly been cured of their affliction with apparent ease, simply because of the intervention of one particular person, who inexplicably succeeds when many others have failed.

Countless people have tried and failed to explain this most valuable of therapies, each with their own particular theory, but unable to validate them to the world's satisfaction. Some people believe spiritual healing is a direct act of God, whereby healing spiritual energies are directed to the afflicted via a third party, others believe spiritual healing is not so much a spiritual miracle, but merely a by-product of our electro-magnetic field.

This second theory can certainly be validated to a degree, in that we are all controlled by electrical impulses via our brain and central nervous systems, and some people do indeed have far greater electrical energy than others. It is this energy which spiritual sceptics claim, allows healers to influence the nervous systems of others to positive effect.

Others believe spiritual healing is an auto-suggestive response whereby the afflicted person can somehow override the effects of their illness by believing that they are cured even if they haven't been physically. It is indeed true that we can in some cases cure illness by self-determination, or cured of some conditions as a result of being hypnotised. This explanation does not apply in all cases though. Whatever the theory, the fact remains that some healers do heal and so they do have a very important place even today with all the modern medicines and surgical techniques we have available.

Spiritual healers work in a very wide range of ways, and at many different locations. Some work in religious institutions, either alone or in a group, whilst others work in clinics or visit people in their own homes individually. (They also work in groups on occasion too). The methods they use to treat people can vary greatly. In the main they use three basic methods, two of which involve direct healing where they are present in the room with you; in the other case they use distance healing methods, which although distant can be just as effective in outcome.

Where healers are working on their patients directly, the patient will be required to either lie down on a bed or therapists' couch, or else sit upright in a chair. Having discussed with the person seeking help, their particular ailment and its repercussions, the healer or healers will then adopt one of two procedures. Either the healer or healers will place their hand or hands on the affected area to be treated, or else, if the person receiving healing is seated, the healer or healers will rest their hands lightly on a person's shoulders, or in some cases will lightly cup their hands over the patient's scalp.

In other cases the healer or healers will carry out a pass, gently moving their hands over the person undergoing treatment; not making physical contact with the person who is the subject of the healing session, but holding their hands flat at a distance of one or two inches away from them.

Very often with both types of treatment the person who is receiving healing can feel something happening. Where direct contact is made, the person who is receiving healing, can often feel a great warmth coming from the healers hands, and down into the affected area of their illness. Where healers' work indirectly, passing their hand over their subject, the person receiving the healing more often than not feels a strange tingling sensation while the healer is working on them.

Sadly not all healers can physically get to meet up with those they are trying to help, either because of distance between them, or because of a particularly heavy caseload, none the less healing therapy can still be administered. In these cases, distance - or absent healing as it is more commonly known - is administered by the healer. If the healer has met the person they are trying to heal once or twice, they will visualise them, or in some cases they will work from a photograph or an object belonging to the person they are trying to help.

Some healers work for free, whilst others charge for their services. Much will depend upon their circumstances. Many healers also practice as physical therapists as well in one context or other and will give healing free of charge during their normal routine, whilst others work as full-time healers. The issue of charging for healing causes great difficulty to most religious healers, since in the main they are merely passing on a God-given gift and are not truly the originator of the product.

There are some however who having decided to work full time, have decided to work on a set fee basis, which can sadly result in cases of serious abuse where fraudsters copy such practices. This being the case, you should therefore be very careful when consulting a healer and discuss their charges beforehand, and when consulting a fee-charging healer, be sure to take up independent testimonials beforehand. That said however, it is important to realise that full-time healers are just like the rest of us, they cannot live on fresh air.

Like the rest of us they have to feed and clothe both themselves and their families, and also meet their financial liabilities as well, and so there are indeed good reasons that some charge a set fee for their services.

To get round this difficult moral dilemma, most reputable healers work on a donations principle based upon what their patients can afford to give them.

Reiki therapy

Reiki therapy is in itself a type of healing therapy which dates back over 2500 years (possibly originating in Tibet), with the modern form of this therapy largely being made popular as a result of the work of a Japanese exponent called Ursi Sensai, though others likewise claim to have made this therapy what it is today with their own versions of this therapy.

Reiki therapists work in a same way to spiritual healers using a very wide range of techniques including music, colour and visualisation therapies, in order to restore harmony to our bodies. Much will depend upon the reiki therapist's background as to which methods of treatment they employ. As with most other "complementary" therapists they work on a set fee basis though some will work on a donations principle as well.

HORMONAL BALANCING THERAPIES

Music and colour therapy

Music and colour therapies are designed to balance our hormonal system and are widely used by both orthodox and "alternative" practitioners alike, both in a physical and psychological context. Many eminent psychoanalysts use colour tests and various colour schemes, both to assess and to treat their patients. It has been found for example that colour schemes in psychiatric wards can and frequently do have great influence in depression or hyperactivity, thus making them a very valuable therapeutic tool.

As a general rule it has been found that the brighter the colour (i.e. red and yellow for example) the more stimulated we become, whereas greens and pastel colours tend to relax us. Darker colours such as grey or black tend to make us very depressed (hence the saying, a black mood).

In respect to colour analysis tests themselves, some practitioners use coloured cards whilst others have bottles of coloured dye which you are required to select in order of preference.

In some cases, a therapist will recommend certain visual images to their patient, or some kind of art therapy using such things as airbrushes or conventional painting techniques.

As with colours, music can be used for therapeutic purposes too. The various speeds and pitches of music can likewise make a considerable difference to us emotionally. More often than not, music therapy is used on a self-help basis as most of us can testify to, either in respect to our listening to, or in some cases physically composing and playing pieces of music.

Crystal healing therapy

Crystal therapy has been widely used since man first walked on the earth, with rocks and stones being greatly prized and valued, not just because of the precious metals which many contain, i.e. gold, tin, copper etc, but also because of their supposedly therapeutic and curative properties.

Today's crystal therapies probably have their origins in North America, with the native Indians being fervent advocates of such therapy even today. In therapeutic terms, crystal therapy can be used in a very wide range of ways, with a great many theories and practices in existence as to how we should use the various precious rocks and stones.. Some people interpret their healing properties in a visual context, with each coloured stone having specific qualities. Others interpret the stones as having a positive life-force of their own which they give off. By far the most prized of stones being quartz and rose quartz, which are believed to have very positive benefits for us in both physical and mental terms (also spiritually).

Because therapists use crystals in many different ways, it is not possible to give precise details in respect to treatment methods. Very often they are used as an additional treatment by many therapists, either to be held by a patient, admired, or used as a focussing tool for inspiration, by either the therapist, or the patient in their home environment.

Visualisation therapy

Visualisation like other emotional therapies works by influencing our hormonal system to positive effect. This is something we all know only too well, in that if we think about pleasant things we feel good about ourselves and life is somehow easier, whereas if we focus upon something bad or upsetting, then we can suddenly find life very uncomfortable.
    Although we are all well aware of these facts it can be very difficult to channel our thoughts in a positive way, and so we can on occasion need the help of a third party, as in cases of severe depression for example. In these circumstances we often need a positive distraction of some kind to lift our spirits. Visualisation therapy can be particularly beneficial in these cases, because unlike similar drug related therapies, there is no risk of overdose, or side effects (see also the meditation information in the self-help section of this book).
    Visualisation therapists can use a very wide range of visualisation depending upon their particular background, some require the patient to focus on particular colours, whilst others give storyline scenarios, either realistic or surreal, often accompanied by a backup tape for home use. Others use graphic images in artistic form and will ask a patient to describe what they are seeing or feeling when they look at a particular visualisation, then counsel their patient accordingly

Yoga

As a method of relaxation yoga is well known, but in actual fact yoga can be and frequently an invaluable therapy too. Sadly when most people visualise yoga they tend to think of an Indian guru sitting in a prayer mat, and therefore think of yoga as just another religion rather than a therapy in itself.

In a therapeutic capacity, yoga does in fact have a very wide range of applications, both mentally and also physically. Indeed health is the main philosophy of this most valuable and ancient practice. Besides clearing our minds and helping to make us much more resilient in respect to stress, yoga can also prove invaluable in respect to personal discipline and body posture as well.

The downside to this therapy however lies in the fact that it requires a tremendous amount of self-discipline, both in respect to setting aside time to practice, and also, in being able to physically shut down your conscious thought processes. For beginners, yoga is therefore best practised in group sessions to start off with. Yoga postures are also extremely beneficial to us in helping with or overall posture and in re-tensioning our muscles too

COUNSELLING THERAPIES

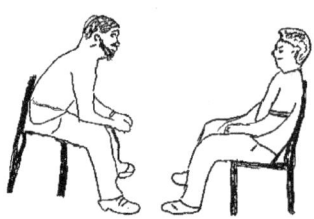

General counselling

General counselling deals primarily with people's feelings, both in respect to themselves, and on occasion their feeling towards others. General counsellors are on hand to help us cope with issues such as bereavement, redundancy, post-traumatic stress (following a crime or serious accidents etc).
    For the most part counsellors are there to listen rather than to physically intervene in any problems we may have. Whilst it is true that we all have friends or relatives we can turn to, it can be a great help talking to someone not directly involved in our situation and who is completely neutral.
    In some instances, a counsellor may be able to help by having useful contact numbers at their fingertips, or if our situation is a desperate one, they may be able to arrange a meeting with someone who can help us in a direct physical way to find housing or some kind of financial assistance. (The Citizens Advice Bureau being a prime example of such a service). In a good many cases such services are run by charities and so they are free, though they do have running costs, and so some kind of donation should be offered them where possible.

Stress consultants

Stress Consultants more often than not work on a private practice basis and service large companies and their workforce. They do also work in clinics and from offices as well, so they are available to the general pubic too. Unlike counsellors, stress consultants do generally have an interventionist policy where individuals consult them, either by administering a physical relaxation treatment of some kind, or by providing a psychological relaxation tool for them to use at home, such as a relaxation recording of some type. (Much will depend upon the therapists' background and range of professional skills in this respect).

After questioning their patients at length, stress consultants may on occasion highlight the options available in respect to a given situation; or suggest lifestyle changes which will help their patients. At the end of the day however, they will only be suggestions, and it will be up to the patient to consider these and their full implications thoroughly, before acting on any suggestions.

Dieticians

More often than not dieticians are allied to general practices and hospitals, though they do also work privately in clinics or as consultants to sports associations as well.

Most dieticians in general practice offer a non-interventionist service, and are there merely to give you support and guidance as appropriate in respect to calorie intake and foodstuffs to avoid or to start consuming as an alternative to your usual meals. Where private practitioners are concerned they can use a wide range of methods to assist you depending upon their particular skills. Some therapists for example will offer a physical treatment programme in respect to aromatherapy massage, which can be particularly effective when treating obesity, whilst others will offer certain types of supplement, or in some cases, diuretic (fluid expulsion chemicals) will be prescribed. Where such chemicals are prescribed however they should only be used in conjunction with supervision with a qualified medical practitioner, since complications can arise when taking such chemicals.

RELATIONSHIP COUNSELLING THERAPIES

Relationship counselling/mediation

These days mediation is a very widely used tool where established relationships get into trouble, particularly in respect to parent/children relationships, or (more commonly) sexual partnerships. In these cases it takes very highly trained and skilled therapists to sort out such conflicts.

In most cases, both of those involved will be required to attend a regular meeting and will be seen both together and also separately. In order to help those in conflict, the therapist will need to hear both sides of any argument and be seen to be neutral, this being the case most relationship therapists will seek to stimulate calm dialogue between both parties so that they both know where they stand.

Sadly most conflicts are born of misunderstanding where one party fails to get across their feelings to another in an effective way, or fails to realise that their behaviour is damaging the relationship. Being very aware of this fact, generally speaking, the therapists will seek to provide a platform so that the less dominant of the two parties can express themselves fully. Once this has been achieved, both parties will then be able to decide clearly upon the way forward for both of them.

Sex therapists

Sex therapists (relationship counsellors) work in pretty much the same way as I've just described in respect to relationship counselling. Contrary to the appearance of their title, more often not therapy sessions concentrate upon the feelings of those concerned, and the need for adequate foreplay and mutual understanding, rather than focussing on physical activity. During counselling sessions, reference is frequent made in respect to educational reading/video educational matter (of which there is a wealth of material available).

PSYCHOTHERAPY

Behavioural therapists

Behavioural therapists work in many different ways, using a wide range of techniques, to treat conditions such as depression, hyperactivity, anger management, alcoholism, drug addiction and compulsions to steal. Such therapists work either on a one to one basis, or in some cases a group therapy situation. Very often when working on a one to one basis with a client, behavioural therapists will use cognitive behaviour therapy. Those seeking such therapy will generally be encouraged to look at themselves and behaviour in detail and make up a list of positive attributes or goals. After discussing any relevant issues, the person undergoing therapy will then be told to focus on those points frequently in a home situation. This will be done either by reciting from a formal list drawn up during the therapy session or by quoting certain positive statements in a self affirming way similar to self- hypnosis.

Group therapy

Group therapy can be a particularly helpful medium for those undergoing therapy in that they have the support of those around them and can see that they are not alone with their particular problem. Very often people who attend the sessions are required to give a background to their particular problem and physically share their experiences with the other members of the group. The therapist sits amongst them prompting the participants as appropriate, whilst they share their triumphs, and failures.

Hypnotherapy

As with most other "complementary" therapies, hypnotherapists rely upon natural healing methods to help their clients. In their case, they use relaxation to balance the mind and body and to correct any patterns of behaviour which are detrimental to their patient's well-being.

Hypnotherapy is in itself a very complex form of one to one therapy, which can and does, treat a very wide range of conditions and behavioural problems, most of which have failed to respond to conventional therapies, because they stem from sub-conscious forces of one type or another. Conditions such as bedwetting in children, insomnia, impotence, nail-biting, blushing, stuttering, phobias, depression, temper tantrums, shyness, inferiority complexes, cigarette addictions and overeating compulsions, are all typical examples where hypnotherapy can be of great benefit. All respond well to hypnotherapy and have a good success rate, though it does depend upon the patient's degree of co-operation.

In order to carry out this type of therapy, the therapist puts their client into a light hypnotic trance, then either asks them to recall past experiences, or else makes positively phrased suggestions to them whilst they are under hypnosis.

As with most other therapies, hypnotherapy has a long pedigree which can be traced back to the pharaohs and beyond, being widely used around the world, both for religious and medical purposes. Here in the western world our knowledge and familiarity of hypnosis stems largely from the work of Franz Anton Mesmer who studied the phenomena in great detail during the 1700's.

In order to understand the principles behind hypnotherapy you first have to understand the scientific term "cause and effect" whereby there must always be a cause or reason for a phenomena.

As with most health problems, to succeed you must first find/treat their cause, before any symptoms will disappear. In some cases this can take a great deal of effort, for both ourselves, and the therapist involved, because like our bodies, our minds and thought processes are very complex in nature.

Probably the clearest proof of this can be seen in a physical sense through our bodily movements/functions. Firstly we have conscious actions, physical movement of our limbs etc, which occur through a conscious decision on our part; secondly we also have an automatic system of physical movement if you think about it. We do not for example will our heart or digestion to work, they have a will of their own, and will work at night when we are asleep, just the same as if we were awake.

Just as the body works on two levels, so also does the mind, in that our thought processes also work on two levels (i.e. the conscious and the unconscious). Our conscious thought processes for example, are those where we physically think things through and act directly as a result of conscious reasoning; our unconscious thought processes on the other hand serve as a constant backup at a subconscious level, planning our everyday routine, and supervising our thoughts generally.

When treating people, therapists take these subconscious thought processes into account, just as much as they do our physical symptoms, for they know only too well that emotional conflicts often have a great bearing upon any physical conditions we may present.

As we all know, life's conflicts can on occasion leave us terribly scarred (especially those arising from childhood experiences). It is often these experiences which are at the root of any adult behavioural problems we may have.

Fortunately as adults we are able to deal with most of life's conflicts; and, given the opportunity to think about them, can work them out to a satisfactory conclusion. This is not true in the case of some childhood conflicts however. All of us at some stage in our early years experienced one crisis or another which we were unable to deal with at the time. Because we lacked adult reasoning, we put these on hold so to speak, we conveniently forgot about them. We may have been involved in an accident, been a victim of, or committed some minor crime which we feel very guilty about on a subconscious level for example. In the case of some of these experiences, they were most unpleasant and carried with them a great deal of emotion, these we put under lock and key. They became what therapists technically call repressions, and it is these memories which hypnotherapists help their clients to recall.

It is the job of your nearest hypnotherapist to uncover these forgotten secrets, so that we can recall them and deal with them by way of adult reasoning, so that we can put them behind us and get on with our lives. By far the most effective way of achieving this is to use therapeutic hypnosis. Once a client has become fully relaxed and has entered the state of hypnosis, the therapist is then able to tap into their sub-conscious mind, where the disturbing repressions are stored. Slowly but surely each repression will come to the surface and be released.

When I make reference to therapeutic hypnosis I am talking of a very pleasant, relaxed state. Some therapists call it, conscious hypnosis; a term which describes the phenomena perfectly. Far from being under a spell and at the mercy of the therapist as some might assume, the patient is to all intense and purposes, fully conscious, and co-operates fully at their own pace and will. Surprising though it may seem, the patient under hypnosis is not just aware of their environment, they are even more so than they would normally be.

In this deep relaxed state with their eyes closed they can hear the everyday sounds around them, they can hear the traffic outside, they can even smell the air in the room more effectively. Should the person undergoing therapy feel uncomfortable and wish to, they could open their eyes, or get up from the couch, without any trouble at all. Whilst a patient's state of relaxation may be very deep, the level of hypnotic trance is in effect very shallow for obvious reasons. If the person concerned were in too deep a state of hypnosis, they would not be in a position to carry out their task of recalling the past.

Having made these statements, you are probably wondering what the difference between therapeutic hypnosis and the everyday waking state are, well firstly (as I've already indicated) under therapeutic hypnosis we are inclined to be more relaxed and so as a result, our processes of recall will be considerably improved.

We will in most cases for example, be able to remember many events from our third or fourth year of age, which we had consciously forgotten. (In some cases it is possible to go back even further). It has also been found that in the hypnotic state, one is much freer of guilt, and so miss-deeds or painful memories are therefore far more likely to come to the surface than in conventional analysis, analysis which can, and does, take many months to establish the same bond between client/therapist that is required.

Whilst the patients are in this state, the therapist lets them piece together events from the past, until that elusive troublesome memory or series of memories come to the surface. When full transference has been attained, a patient will re-experience the event which was repressed, just as they did when it originally happened. Once this has taken place, the therapist concerned simply has to tie up any loose ends, and bid the client farewell, to live life as they see fit.

It is not the hypnotherapists' job to judge others actions, or to advise them, but simply to guide their patient, to a full state of self awareness. The insight the patient gets into themselves, comes from themselves; and they make the decisions as regards their future. All the therapists have done is to help them put the past well and truly behind them.

As I am sure you will now appreciate, many repressions are of a disturbing or an embarrassing nature and so a very strong bond between client and therapist is required. It is only when this bond has been established that the repression or repression's will come to light - and be released.

Like many other psychotherapies, hypnotherapy relies upon a special state of unity with the therapist which I have just mentioned in respect to transference, whereby the client; through the induced state of calm and personal dynamics of the client/therapist relationship, recalls emotions as well as the events from the past. In the case of repressed memories, this is essential, for until the emotion is released along with the incident, no proper relief can be attained. The process usually takes between six to eight weeks to develop fully, though in some cases it can take longer, and largely depends upon the client's degree of co-operation.

As with most psychological therapies, the benefit a patient will get, very much depends upon their personal input into the process. With analytical hypnotherapy that process is a very simple one, all a patient has to do is to lie still and quiet on a couch and simply answer a therapists' questions, as truthfully as they can. Whilst some questioning may be of a directly personal nature, more often than not a therapist will rely upon a process called, " free association" in that a patient will simply be asked to clear their mind of all immediate thoughts and say the first thing, or things which comes into their heads. The key word here is "free" however: to be effective such memories must be free and not held back or forced by ourselves.

Whilst this may seem a strange procedure, both the patient and the therapist will know that they are looking for something, something hidden deep in their sub-conscious past. Once the patient has come up with a seemingly trivial memory, or series of memories, the therapist will help them to enlarge upon that subject, by asking carefully targeted questions, prompting them as necessary. The patient will eventually discover a situation which has influenced their behaviour since its occurrence, and will be able to rationalise that situation as an adult and neutralise its effects so that it cannot do them any more harm.

Some people doubt they can be hypnotised, this is however a total misconception on their part, since all persons pass through the hypnotic state at least twice a day. Firstly we do so when we awaken in the morning, and secondly, when we go to sleep at night; though of course the depth of hypnotic induction does vary from person to person; but please be assured, all people are capable of entering the hypnotic state at some point.

Since there is no such thing as a hypnotised feeling, the person under hypnosis is unlikely to realise they have entered hypnosis itself. It is just a pleasant, calm, peaceful sort of feeling, which the therapists aim to utilise to the client's full advantage.

In almost all cases, hypnotherapists are able to assist the patients that come to them, so that their problems are resolved speedily, and most importantly permanently, thus relieving them of a lifetime's unnecessary stress in the process. There are of course some individuals that therapists would not try to hypnotise, namely those of a very low I.Q, people who are heavily drugged, or in a drunken state for example, but apart from these people, anyone who is of sound mind can be hypnotised.

As well as normal analytical therapy under hypnosis, there is another service which some therapists offer called suggestion therapy. This can be very useful where a patient wants to attain a certain weight or stop smoking etc. Under these circumstances, a patient will utilise the power of hypnosis to amend any negative aspects of their behaviour, for it is known that people are far more responsive to suggestion when under hypnosis (as the stage hypnotist is only too willing to demonstrate).

It is possible, with carefully worded statements, to correct a person's bad habits through suggestion therapy in some cases; provided they are not too serious. Such treatments can prove very effective under the right circumstances. They do however have their limitations, particularly in respect of the more severe cases of obesity, cigarette addictions and alcoholism. Very often a therapist will recommend direct analytical therapy in these cases.

Hypnotherapists know from experience that serious disorders such as obesity, cigarette addictions and alcoholism are often of the oral satisfaction type, and that there is generally a root cause for such behaviour; which must be traced before any long-term benefit can be attained. Under these circumstances, a patient will be issued with a relevant suggestion therapy tape, merely to reinforce their treatment sessions, rather than it providing the cure; that said, most people will respond favourably to suggestion therapy in its own right and so it is always worth trying first, before embarking upon more costly analytical methods.

Anyone wishing to try suggestion therapy does need to be very careful who they approach, for carried out by a person not properly qualified to conduct this form of therapy, could result in their problem being made far worse. When contemplating such therapy, it is best to ask around, and choose a therapist who has been recommended by others through personal experience, preferably someone who has a proven track record, and is registered with a professional association of some kind.

During a treatment program, therapists sometimes use what are called subliminal sound messages, whereby their voices are speeded up and raised to a frequency above the range of our conscious hearing. This allows them to use carefully worded phrases to relax a client, or to help their client correct a bad habit which they are trying to overcome at a subconscious level. Because of the way such phrases are delivered, a therapist is able to bypass the critical faculty of their client's conscious mind. Any comments made in this way will go directly to their client's sub-conscious, thus ensuring that any instructions/suggestions will be taken at face value, rather than be judged, and possibly discarded by our conscious thought processes.

Subliminal sound messages are sometimes dubbed onto a music cassette or digital recording disk of some kind and played amongst background music during the treatment session. In some cases therapists will issue these recordings to their patients so that they can use them in their home environment to fortify their treatment. In such cases a therapist will generally recommend that they are played, say ten times, over a fourteen-day period, and then once a week until the treatment programme has been completed.
Probably the best way to illustrate the benefit of this therapy is through the following case history:

Think about a young man with an inferiority complex for example, he feels totally useless, he doesn't really know why; he just does. In later life he finds he hasn't got the confidence to get a decent job; he's certain he is going to make some sort of stupid mistake which would undermine his confidence even further, so when a decent job comes his way, he doesn't even bother to apply. He is certain if he got the job he would make some stupid mistake and get dismissed.

The same sort of attitude prevails as regards life partners; he is so shy and bashful that when he meets someone he finds attractive, he can't find the words to even speak to them; he doesn't know why he just can't. He in his wisdom goes to his doctor and if he is lucky, he will get a referral a psychiatrist or conventional analyst. Despite wholehearted effort on everybody's part, it is highly unlikely that the cause of his attitude problem will be established by analysis alone. To be so powerful an attitude problem, it must have been a very shameful or embarrassing experience which would have created this negative attitude in the person concerned.

The term cause and effect certainly applies in this case. There must be a reason for his self discrediting attitude. As you will now appreciate, what ever happened to that person will have succumbed to repression (i.e. been forgotten by his conscious mind). No matter how trivial it appears to us with adult reasoning, when whatever happened to that person happened, it was dealt with by childhood logic. To him it was a major catastrophe, which had to be put under lock and key in his sub-conscious; where even he as an adult couldn't find it.

Fortunately hypnotherapy can help in such cases. Hypnotherapists know from experience that by using their particular skills, they can tap into that person's sub-conscious and help them find the incident which has blighted their life until now. By reawakening that person's memory, hypnotherapists can release them from their pitiful existence. Once that person has re-experienced their original mishap and seen it through adult eyes, they are then able to put it behind them and can live a full and enjoyable life from then on; their ghost will finally be laid to rest.

Whilst it's not practical to discuss therapists' individual fees; regardless of cost, in most cases they are more than reasonable when you consider the results they achieve. Take the case of that young man with the inferiority complex for example; the cost of his treatment was minimal in comparison to the freedom which he now has.

Many therapists offer an initial consultation free of charge to discuss any particular problem or problems. This is particularly useful, since it gives patients the chance to meet a practitioner before they commit themselves to therapy. In many cases a strong bond is established at that very first meeting and therapy commences soon afterwards.

In some cases, self-hypnosis can be used (see self-hypnosis, pages 138-141). Whilst being a considerably cheaper option, tremendous self-control/willpower can be required if such an option is to be successful however.

DIAGNOSTIC TOOLS

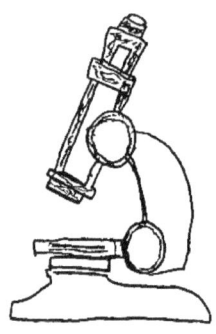

Kirlian photography

Throughout history there have been reports of people giving off spiritual auras in that they appeared to glow with some sort of special aura. Many healers in the past have claimed that they could see and treat disorders according to such auras. In a great many cases however, auras have been put down to the person's electro-magnetic field, rather than their own spiritual blueprint. Thanks to modern technology it is now possible to record such auras in a physical format.

Kirlian photography is named after Semyon and Valentina Kirlian who developed a high frequency photographic technique to monitor people's auras during the 1970's. Since then the technique has been widely adopted across the world, particularly by spiritual healers. Sadly this valuable diagnostic tool, has like so many therapies, suffered as a result of bad publicity, because unsubstantiated diagnostic claims have been made in respect to this relatively new and exciting medium by some therapists.

In most cases practitioners will take a high frequency photograph of the patient's hand or hands. Once processed the image or images will show varying coloration or shading around the periphery of the limb or limbs photographed. From these images, the therapist or healer will assess your energy flows and any imbalances which have shown up, then will either seek to treat you themselves, (depending upon their qualifications), or else will refer you to a more appropriate therapist for your particular condition.

Iridology

Iridology is a therapy principle involving examination of the eyes in order to assess the state of health of the patient. As a "diagnostic tool," iridology is widely used by a great many practitioners (including orthodox medical practitioners), since it is known that a great many conditions can be correctly diagnosed through studying the iris and surrounding tissue. The potential risk of heart attacks and strokes for example, can often be identified by studying the eye and surrounding blood vessels. As we all know, it is only too easy to see people's lifestyles through their eyes on occasion too.
   The therapy itself originated over 100 years ago, being developed by an American doctor (Dr Bernard Jensen) and has undergone much adaptation over the years, with photographic detail being used for assessment by many modern practitioners.

Once a photograph has been taken of the patient's eyes, the patients' health status is then assessed using a comprehensive chart, mapping each area of the eye, dividing it up in sections corresponding to the patients physical body layout. (This is done in a similar way to which reflexologists work with their charts). Such things as flecks and areas of cloudiness on the photographs are then cross-referenced with the Iridology charts. These give the therapist an insight in respect to the origins of any health disorders so that they may then be treated, either by the therapist directly (depending upon their qualifications) or else by the most suitable practitioner for the patient's particular condition.

Dowsing

Dowsing is diagnostic technique generally used by spiritual healers. In most cases the person carrying out this type of technique will use a precious stone of some kind suspended from a chain.

Depending upon the circumstances for the diagnosis, the healer will use a chart, or series of charts, with details of possible causes, or treatments for a particular condition. Having held the dowsing tool (pendulum) over the charts for a short while, the suspended stone or crystal will often sway; either backwards and forwards, or rotate in a circle, over one particular area of the chart. This gives the healer possible indications as to the origins and treatments for the condition they are required to treat.

In most cases this procedure will be carried out by the healer in private, once the patient has left the surgery. Whilst such methods may at face value seem somewhat hap-hazard or bizarre, they are sometimes very accurate, and so they do indeed work.

As to the reason for this - whilst the bulk of dowsers would suggest divine assistance, a great many sceptics point to out that most healers are also very experienced and well qualified therapists. Many suspect that the dowsing tool can in fact be influenced by the slightest movement of the dowser's hand, which implies to the sceptics that the process is in fact a trick of the dowser's sub-conscious, whereby they are using their vast knowledge of health issues and potential signs in an unconscious way.

Allergy testing

Allergy testing is a service widely available within the "complementary" healthcare service. Equipment and treatment practices can vary widely. In all cases, diagnosis is generally pretty accurate. Most diagnostic equipment involves small quantities of possible irritants (i.e. food, or household debris/products) used in conjunction with a low voltage electrical circuit. More often than not a patient is asked to hold an electrode, or one is placed at certain points on our body (i.e. our hands, wrists feet etc), this will make up a complete circuit. A wide range of foods and other matter will be included somewhere within that circuit, with each item of matter being tested in turn (one item at time).
    Sensitivity responses are usually measured via a meter reading, or in some cases by our pulse. Probably the most widely known of such testing devices is the vega test devised by a Dr Schimmel. Whilst these tests are quite painless physically (unlike scratch tests carried out by some hospitals), they can be extremely expensive in some cases.

Generally speaking where specific allergies are identified the offending allergens should be avoided for a period of time (possibly on a permanent basis, in the case of many household products). Where house dust proves to be the main offender, there are a whole host of measures we can take. Besides hoovering and dusting regularly, it is also important to change our bedding on a frequent basis. Fortunately there are now a great many furnishing/bedding materials which are specifically designed to reduce the risk of dust mites (often the main source of house dust allergens). In view of their availability it is therefore a good idea to purchase and use such products where such allergies occur.

Where offending foods are of an essential nature (i.e. dairy produce, wheat, meat, etc), they should slowly be re-introduced into our diet over a period of time, with our health being closely monitored in respect to any ill effects which re-introduction may cause.

Before taking dietary advice, it's generally best to research a practitioners' background (seeking references where necessary). Ideally where dietary advice is given by such practitioners, it's best to get a second opinion from a qualified dietician or doctor since long-term exclusion of certain foodstuffs can in some cases be injurious to our health.

SELF HELP SECTION

SELF HELP

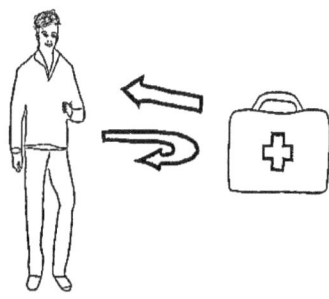

In this section of the guide I will concentrate upon things which we can do for ourselves, either in respect to treatment, pain relief, or in the case of our diets and stress, measures we can take to protect ourselves from ill health.

With the vast array of "alternative" therapies available to us nowadays, it's little wonder that some people opt to treat themselves, especially since time is so precious to us these days. In some cases we can find it very difficult making appointments to see doctors or specialists because they are so busy, or else we likewise are too busy to visit them.

Off the Shelf and Internet Products

Whilst there are a great many "alternative" treatments and health-food supplements available for us to buy at local health-food and drug stores, they can when misused, bring about more complex health disorders, and so we should be very wary of them. Besides asking advice from those selling such remedies, it is also a good idea to read up as much as you can prior to using them. Above all, you should always take time to study product packaging for details in respect to dosage and warnings.

PAIN RELIEF

Sadly pain is something we all experience from time to time. In some cases pain can prevent us from sleeping, working, or simply going about our normal daily routines (i.e. migraines, arthritis etc). Besides being extremely uncomfortable, pain can therefore inconvenience us greatly. It is however important to realise that pain occurs for a reason. Pain is a warning system that there is something wrong, or that we are in danger of some kind.

Whilst there are a wide range of options available to us, i.e. painkillers etc, its important to identify the cause of your pain before using them, since masking pain can be an extremely dangerous thing to do in some cases (i.e. where severe stomach/chest pains or headaches occur suddenly).

In most cases, where pain occurs, it's best to consult a qualified medical practitioner/doctor (especially where pain or discomfort last for more than a few hours).

Where your situation has been assessed by qualified persons, you are then in a better position to employ pain relief methods. In most cases supervising practitioners will prescribe pain relief of some sort themselves. Sadly where long-term conditions such as arthritis occur however, we can often find that we have to fend for ourselves in most cases, hence the inclusion of this particular section within this guide.

Fortunately besides conventional man made drugs i.e. painkillers such as asprin, paracetamol etc, there are also a wide range of other options open to us in respect to self-help pain relief, many of which I am about to outline. Not only do we have the option of acupressure (as outlined on pages 43 - 44) we also have a whole host of other equally valid options to choose from as well (depending upon our condition).

In some cases, people find electronic equipment useful, either in the form of ultrasonic/infrasonic massage equipment, both of which work by sending small electronic pulses deep into our tissue where normal massage would prove ineffective. This form of therapy is often used to great effect by professional sports therapists, though there are a wide range of similar products designed for the domestic market.

As well as direct massage based equipment electronic, pulse units of the T.E.N.S (transcutaneous nerve stimulation) variety are also widely available. Unlike infrasound/ultrasound, these work to sedate/stimulate our nervous system, rather than massage affected areas. As well as being widely available for domestic use, such equipment is also used in orthodox medicine sometimes too, to treat conditions where pain occurs repeatedly.

Electronic equipment is not suitable for use by everybody however; where people have a heart pacemaker for example, such equipment could in some cases be affected by a medical electronic device of the sort I've just described. Such technology is not advisable during pregnancy or where someone has epilepsy either. As with oral medicines/healthfood remedies etc, it is essential that qualified professional advice is sought before purchasing or using such equipment, with all product packaging being read thoroughly before use.

Recently magnet therapy has become very popular in respect to pain relief and indeed can prove very effective (especially where arthritic conditions prevail). Whilst we are not entirely sure as to how such products work, it is widely believed that they work via our blood (in a similar way to an air ioniser) to restore harmony to our body tissue. As with electronic equipment however, magnet based products should not be used where one has a pacemaker.

Possibly a safer alternative in this respect would be copper bracelets. They have been traditionally used to great effect all through history, to relieve conditions such as rheumatism and arthritis; though again medical supervision should be undertaken as copper may in some cases prove detrimental in respect to allergic reactions, unintended absorption via the skin etcetera.

HOME PHYSIOTHERAPY TREATMENT

Strains and sprains

In respect to strains and sprains, there is a great deal we can do to relieve these conditions ourselves if we act fast enough. In a good many cases we have pushed ourselves too far, either as an athlete, or through overexertion during our working day, in a leisure pursuit or sporting activity.

In both cases, the way in which we deal with injuries is crucial in respect to their long-term outcome in most cases. Sadly the body tends to over-react when strains and sprains occur, which can, and often does, result in painful swelling. This is one area where we can do something positive to help ourselves. We can for example administer first aid to the organ we have damaged, just as we would if we had cut ourselves and were suffering blood loss.

Whilst we cannot see any signs of physical action, it is almost certain that following a strain or sprain the affected area will become overrun with fluids if we don't do something. Just as we do with a cut, it is therefore necessary to cool the affected area by means of a cold flannel (or as is often used, a bag of frozen peas, wrapped in a damp towel/flannel). You should then bandage the affected area (but not too tightly; just tight enough so that it is firmly bound but still comfortable and won't cut off your blood supply), in order to prevent the inevitable swelling which is likely to occur if left untreated.

There are also anaesthetic sprays that we can use to treat the affected areas, though these can do more harm than good in some cases. By anaesthetising the area it is not possible to gauge the intensity of an injury; this being so, in some cases we may be inclined to use an injured organ when we should be resting it.

It is very important to realise that pain occurs for a very important reason, i.e. to warn us that body tissue is damaged in some way, so that we can take action to repair it. If we carry on using those affected organs then we are likely to run the risk of doing permanent damage to them.

Having administered first aid, it is important to rest those areas that are injured, though in some cases such as shoulder, hip and leg injuries this can be very difficult in respect to work/family commitments etc. The main thing to remember in these circumstances is that the first forty-eight hours are crucial to your recovery. It is far better to sacrifice those forty-eight hours, than lose far more time long-term as a result of prolonged or secondary injuries (which can easily occur where we overuse our other limbs or muscles, in order to protect those we have damaged). Once forty-eight hours have elapsed, you can then assess your injury in respect to its severity.

In most cases it's a good idea to seek professional advice, especially so if you are a professional athlete, or your work requires you to use the affected limb. With many physical injuries, (and indeed some painful conditions such as arthritis for example,) it's necessary to undertake supervised exercise. This can prove both very painful, and exhausting in some instances. Sadly this can be a price we have to pay if we are to make a full recovery from our condition (or at least retain a reasonable degree of mobility).

Regardless of our choice of action, the same principles apply in all cases in that we must support the area we have damaged so that it can heal properly. Often the best way of doing so is by using some form of elasticated support. In most cases this will allow us to use the affected area when necessary without doing further damage (provided you we are careful).

Where an injury of some sort has occurred, it may be that we can only manage a few painful steps at first, but as time goes by, with perseverance we will find that we can manage a few more, and then a few more. In such cases it's very important to pace ourselves in respect to such exercises however, to set achievable goals, and above all, note the successes of our endeavours (no matter how small), since each step forward is progress, no matter how tiny the step.

DIET AND NUTRITION

Where our diets are concerned, there are plenty of things we can do to protect ourselves health-wise; all require long-term commitment and dedication to the tasks in hand, (i.e. eating a healthy and mixed diet on a permanent basis for example).

Sadly very few of us give sufficient thought to our diets and the long-term implications in respect to our normal diet. What most of us fail to consider is the fact that the food we are eating is not merely fuel as most of us think, the proteins fats etc actually become our bodies within a relatively short space of time. In other words we are what we eat, quite literally. This being the case, it's important that we all eat a balanced diet if we are to remain healthy.

It is also important that we acknowledge that nutritional needs can and do vary greatly from person to person, depending upon their age, lifestyle and metabolism. Being such a crucial component in our lives we cannot afford to be complacent where food intake is concerned. It is therefore important that we all have a basic understanding of the nutritional process and adhere to the rules that have been established over many years, in respect to nutrition and the proven effects any deficiencies will have upon us. Sadly All too many of us are swayed by the wealth of recent trends/theories that abound these days in respect to our nutritional needs, few of which have been proven to be of benefit long-term.

It is also important that we understand a little about the chemical processes involved and why we need to eat certain foodstuffs, or must avoid eating others in large quantities in order to remain healthy so that we can make informed choices for ourselves.

Nutritional components

Foodstuffs come in 3 main categories, fats, carbohydrates and proteins, all of which are essential for our wellbeing. Fats for example provide us with fuel (generally on a short-term basis) they come in two types i.e. saturated fats and unsaturated fats. The second main food group, carbohydrates, provide us with long-term energy. The third dietary group are proteins (the body's main building blocks). Besides these main groups there are other elements which we need, i.e. vitamins minerals and trace elements. Together these various components make up a balanced diet, essential for our wellbeing. (If we lack any of these components we are likely to become ill.)
  As a food group, fats have a very bad reputation, since they can (particularly saturated fats) if consumed to excess, make us very ill/obese; this largely depends upon their type however (a point which many people fail to grasp). The minute people hear the word fat they automatically start to panic, in a good many cases believing that they will automatically get obese if they consume any fatty foodstuffs, which is not necessarily the case. Whilst it is true that eating too many fat rich foods can bring about obesity/illness, they are an essential foodstuff, providing us with both movement and heat energy. Where weight gain is concerned, much depends upon our metabolism and the type of fats we consume, i.e. whether they are predominantly saturated or unsaturated.
  These two types of fat, come from very different sources. Saturated fats come largely from dairy produce and general meat products, whilst unsaturated fats are found in margarine, nuts, cooking oils, fish etc. The principal difference between them being (as their titles suggest), saturated fats come in solid form, unsaturated fats on the other hand occur largely in a liquefied state (with the exception of margarine, which has thickening agents added).

As I've already indicated, whilst saturated fats can provide us with general movement/heat fuel, they can easily put our health at risk if we consume them in too high a dose, because of their tendency to solidify, thus furring/clogging up our arteries. (Where we amass large quantities of physical body fat, this can likewise be bad for us in respect to the strain on our heart and circulatory systems.) Unsaturated fats on the other hand, are far more beneficial, in that whilst they provide us with fuel, they pose less of a health risk than their thicker counterparts.

When calculating our dietary requirements, it is important for us to remember that besides needing fuel for our bodies, we also need a certain amount of fuel for our thought processes too. This is a role which unsaturated fats serve very efficiently, in that they can give us short-term energy but in a safer form.

With both kinds of fat, it's important to monitor them in relation to our intake. Fortunately cream cakes, fatty foods, sugary drinks etc receive much publicity in the press and so we can easily identify them and know when we're eating too many of them. Other food elements do not get so much publicity however (vitamins, minerals, trace elements for example). Also, closely allied to fats, we have carbohydrates; i.e. bread, potatoes, pasta, cereals etc. These foodstuffs likewise provide us with energy but in a more efficient way, and on a long-term basis. Although they are a healthier dietary component than saturated fats they can still bring about undesired weight gain if consumed to excess (the same is true of proteins of course). Whilst the main role of protein lies in respect to the repair of our body tissue, if consumed to excess, then any surplus protein will likewise be converted into fuel and laid down as fat.

Unlike fats/carbohydrates, there are many different types of proteins, all found in different food sources. Of the three main groups, proteins are undoubtedly the most important, since they are the body's building blocks, which physically make up our body tissue. We must therefore ensure that they are consumed in a reasonable quantity. They are found principally in meat, and dairy products, eggs, milk, cheese etc. though they can also be found in cereals nuts and vegetables too. In order to maintain our body tissue to an adequate level, it's important that we consume a wide range of protein rich foods on a regular basis, since each type of protein has different properties, beneficial to certain body organs.

Besides these three main food components, we also need to ensure we get an adequate supply of vitamins, minerals and trace elements too.

Most vitamins work to regulate our metabolism (particularly the vitamin B group). Like proteins, they are obtained from a wide range of food sources, and take many different forms, i.e. vitamin A, B, C, D, E and K, with each group doing different jobs. Some have direct physical roles; vitamin, A for example (found in dairy produce and green vegetables) helps to maintain our hair, skin, sight, teeth etc, whilst vitamin D (found in dairy produce fish oils and margarine) is important for the development and maintenance of our bone structure. Vitamin C is known to be very important in respect to our connective tissue and is believed to play a major role in our immune system too, hence the tendency of many nutritionists to recommend vitamin C rich foods and drinks (containing citrus fruits, i.e. oranges, lemon and blackcurrant) when we are ill.

The vitamin B group is made up of many different vitamins, the main ones being B1 (thiamine), B2 (riboflavin), B5 (pantothenic Acid), B6, B12, biotin, niacin and choline. (The greatest sources of these nutrients being meat and cereal.) Whilst all vitamins are very important, B group vitamins are especially so, in that they are fundamental in our general metabolism, particularly in respect to our blood composition (B6 and 12 in particular, where women's health are concerned). The final two vitamins essential to our wellbeing are vitamins K and E. Vitamin K like the B group vitamins plays a very important part in blood metabolism (found principally in leafy green vegetables), whilst vitamin E is known to be very important in respect to genital tissue and plays a very important part in respect to fertility.

The final set of dietary components consist of minerals and trace elements (generally mineral compounds) which either go to make up our bodies (i.e. calcium, magnesium and phosphorus for example), or else help to balance our bodies (i.e. tissue salts/iodine etc). Most can be easily obtained from dairy products, though salad and vegetables can also provide such nutrients too in some cases, depending upon how and where they are grown, how they are stored and cooked etc.

Besides calcium, magnesium and phosphorus (which go to make up our bone structure and teeth amongst other things), sodium, chlorine, potassium and iodine (which work to balance our body tissue/fluids and glands are also required). We also need ample amounts of iron (which helps with blood metabolism, together with sulphur (which helps our neurological system), plus silicon, which is an important element of our hair, nails etc as well.

Where trace elements are concerned, probably the most important elements are zinc (found, in seafood, vegetables, meat etc) which is a major constituent of our immune system, being required for the growth and repair of body tissue, and selenium (also found in meat, vegetables and cereals), which is needed for red blood cell metabolism

We also need minute traces of aluminium, chromium, copper, and arsenic too if we are to remain healthy; though as with all components mentioned (including vitamins), if consumed in too large a dose, these last components can most definitely prove harmful to us.

Surprising though it may seem, with the exception of highly processed foods, the principle of good foods and bad food is something of a misguided notion. Foods often given publicity (either in a liquid form or in a solid form) of a negative nature, can in fact be very good for us in moderation. Beers wines and spirits for example, each have particular qualities which are of benefit to us. Beers for example may on occasion be beneficial because of their high yeast, vitamin and mineral content, likewise with wine, which is also thought to have valuable anti-oxidant properties too, which can help to reduce the risk of heart complaints. Chocolate is another example. Whilst the sugar in chocolate has always led us to think chocolate products are bad for us, in actual fact cocoa products such as chocolate (particularly dark chocolate) are now believed to have similar anti-oxidant properties to red wine. The key word with all of these foodstuffs however is that of moderation; that particularly applies in the case of alcohol, since some recent studies seem to indicate that any alcohol intake at all might be bad for us.

    As I've already indicated fats are another case in point (particularly saturated fats) in that we need them for energy. That said our nutritional needs are changing quite considerably as we evolve. These days we tend to live a far more sedentary lifestyle. Because we get less exercise these days, we don't need such a high proportion of fatty foods in our diet. Sadly because of our busy lifestyles we are inclined to opt for ready-made convenience meals, which in a good many cases can prove detrimental to our health if consumed to excess (every day), either because they often contain high levels of fat, or because they have high levels of preservatives in them, which are detrimental to us (i.e. salt, processed sugars etc). Fortunately, this latter point has far less relevance these days though because most food producers are working hard to reduce such ingredients in our foods in an attempt to make such meals healthier following much publicity about this potential problem. The same applies to the soft drinks industry too, in that they likewise are working very hard to make previously unhealthy soft drinks more health, reformulating them in a positive way so that we can still enjoy them without them being a potential problem for some people.

    Modern lifestyles and diets also pose a serious health threat to our children too. Sadly we are now starting to see an alarming trend towards obesity in our children. Many of them now spend a large amount of their time sat at computer screens or watching other forms of audio-visual entertainment whilst living almost exclusively on convenience foods. In the past children got far more exercise and so they could easily cope with fatty foods, but now their opportunities for using up fat reserves/calories are greatly reduced. Not only do they play less sport these days, nowadays many are actively discouraged from walking to school or cycling because of perceived dangers. Sadly such attitudes can put them in even greater danger if we are not careful, in that they miss out on much needed opportunities for physical exercise. Lack of physical exercise is something which most of us are guilty of, if we are honest. These days, even for the shortest of journeys we opt to drive. Whilst this may be practical when it is raining, in general terms such behaviour is a recipe for disaster where our metabolism is concerned.

    Not only does exercise provide an opportunity to burn off any excess calories, more importantly, exercise ensures we keep our muscles in shape too. Regular exercise (i.e. walking, cycling etc) also ensures we get adequate supplies of oxygen as well (another major nutrient). Surprising though it may seem, few of us breath properly these days. Because we are in such a hurry (rather than take strong deep breaths as we used to), many of us now take short shallow breaths. This is a practice which in a good many cases deprives us of this essential nutrient (i.e. oxygen). Where we take regular exercise on the other hand, we are often forced to breath more efficiently and so we tend to breath more effectively during our day to day routine, either because of training, or habit.

Personal circumstances

Ideally we should aim for a balanced diet, which includes a full range of nutrients, but which at the same time takes account of our individual circumstances, i.e. our age, workload, general health and metabolic capabilities.
    The nutritional requirements for each individual can and do vary greatly depending upon our particular circumstances and metabolism. In some cases we can process foods very efficiently, or have a physically demanding job or sporting hobby, which will mean that we have less of an issue with high calorie foods in respect to weight gain or potential internal tissue damage. In other cases however, we can find that we need only consume one or two cream cakes and our weight starts to balloon out of control or we put ourselves at risk of ill health internally (i.e. fatty congested arteries which can lead to a heart attack or stroke). One clear and universal situation applies to all though, that being in respect to our age banding requirements. Obviously when we are young we need a full range of nutrients (including saturated fats). As we grow older, we often have to reduce the amount of saturated fats we consume. There is a great difference in respect the needs of men and women too, in that women need to ensure that they have adequate amounts of iron (see women's health pages 114 -116) to cope with their different metabolism. Whilst we are able to store many nutrients within our bodies when we are young; as we age, our storage capacity becomes greatly diminished and so we need to be particularly careful if we are to remain healthy and stay free from colds etc.
    In our younger years good nutritional intake is especially important in order to ensure we grow up to be fit and healthy. We therefore need to ensure that children are given ample amounts of vitamin and mineral rich foods from an early age. (Calcium is particularly important for the development of our bone structure). As well as fresh fruit and vegetables, it is essential that young people consume

plenty of dairy rich foods, such as. milk, cheese etc also a small amount of red meat if it is emotionally acceptable (though this may be difficult where vegan or vegetarian philosophies apply within a household. As a source of nourishment, meat products are particularly important for they are very high in B group vitamins (which are very important for our blood/circulatory system and general metabolism). It is also very important that children get good nutritional advice/education and supervision too, since their whole future (in a health respect) depends upon the food they put into their mouths. Not only will their nutritional intake have a bearing in respect to the time they will live (along with hereditary/circumstantial factors etc), nutritional intake will also have a bearing upon the frequency and disruption to their lives in respect to bouts and types of illness too.

Sadly when it comes to good dietary planning, all too often our conscience (animal welfare issues), time constraints (work etc), or our vanity in respect to fashion (teenage girls in particular), tend to get influence our decisions where nutritional requirements are concerned; animal welfare issues are a prime example. Animal welfare is certainly an issue where we should be concerned, but to deprive ourselves of essential vitamins/minerals in an easy do digest form, can be a risky thing to do in some cases. Regrettably it is a fact of life that we need these particular nutrients and the most effective method of acquiring them is to eat a mix of both animal and plant matter.

This is one sad fact which many would rather ignore, particularly teenage girls who see dairy produce as fattening and who strive desperately to meet the standards set in girl/teen magazines, by fashion models etc. All too often such standards are based on false criteria where role models have had surgery, taken medication or adhered to unhealthy diets, all of which make them look good in the short-term, but which could have grave long-term repercussions when they are no longer in the limelight. Trying to meet such false ideals can seriously put the lives of some impressionable youngsters in great peril, both emotionally and physically, from conditions such as depression, anorexia, surgery compulsions etc, when in actual fact their own bodies are perfectly acceptable as they are. It is therefore important that children realise that body shape is an individual issue. Whilst it is true we can have some influence upon our body shape, at the end of the day our frame/bone structure and hereditary characteristics will determine our visual profile to a large extent. We should therefore be comfortable with our bodies as they are and realise instead that it is our personality which is most important.

Whether or not to live a dairy free/vegetarian lifestyle is of course a matter of personal choice. It should be noted however, that a total vegetarian diet (i.e. a vegan where all meat and dairy produce are excluded) could potentially pose a serious long-term health risk for a wide range of reasons. Firstly, because vegetable sources do not necessarily provide the diversity of proteins we need to keep ourselves healthy, and secondly, it is known that certain cereals can obstruct the nutritional process, effectively blocking the uptake of other essential nutrients.

The greatest risk to our health by following a vegetarian/vegan diet, and omitting all meat and dairy products from our diet, lies in respect to a possible reduction in respect to our intake of B group vitamins and a potentially reduced iron intake (obtained very easily from meat sources). These potential deficiencies could be particularly serious where women are concerned, resulting in conditions such as anaemia, osteoporosis and other more general metabolic disorders. It is also the case that such diets could weaken our immune systems, rendering us liable to more colds and viruses than would generally be the case with a conventional diet. Where we do plan to live a vegetarian lifestyle it is therefore essential that we seek advice from a qualified nutritionist or medical practitioner and consult them on a regular basis. It can likewise be a good idea to have regular checkups with a doctor and have regular blood tests so that any nutritional imbalances can be rectified before any long-term or permanent damage occurs.

Even where we do not pursue a vegetarian/vegan lifestyle, our own general eating preferences can still be a cause of concern in respect to our overall health of course. In some cases, we may have a preference for fatty type foods, say chips, burgers or steak for example. Whilst such preferences may appear to put us at risk of ill health, this needn't be the case. Much depends upon our metabolism, but in all cases there are steps we can take to reduce the risk to our health without necessarily having to forgo such foods. We can for example grill meat so that most of the fat residues drain away. We can also drain off the fat from chips and burgers too, by putting kitchen roll beneath them for a few seconds once we have removed them from our frying device, or alternatively, turn to drier oven chips instead.

Sadly in some cases, the cost and time required to prepare/eat our food can make a considerable difference to us too. Because we lead such busy lives we often tend to eat snack meals of the convenience variety, i.e. crisps, chocolate fast foods etc. Whilst such behaviour may be unavoidable, there are still things we can do in respect to our choices, i.e. buy baked low salt biscuits instead of crisps so that we have a lower fat intake, or buy fried crisp type products etc which state on their packaging that they are lower in fats, salt etc.)

Ideally it would be better if we could buy fresh produce, or grow our own, but sadly all too often, time constraints and financial practicalities tend to block such ideals and so we are forced to make the most of the foodstuffs which come readily to hand.

Nutritional quality

As well as the type of food we consume (i.e. protein, fats, carbohydrates etc), the quality of the food we consume can also make a big difference to our wellbeing. In some cases methods of production/preparation, cooking or storage can damage the nutrients we are hoping to consume. The overcooking of vegetables is a prime example of this, in that whilst vegetables (like other soil grown crops) contain many essential vitamins/minerals these can easily be lost through overcooking, especially where such crops are boiled. This can be clearly illustrated by the fact that during times of war and food shortages, the water used to boil cabbage, spinach etc has been drunk as a type of soup, since it is known that such liquid contains very high levels of iron and other essential nutrients. These days such an approach is not so appealing however, but still the principle holds true in that if we boil crops too much their goodness soon leaches out of them into the surrounding cooking fluids.

    Storage of vegetables is another case in point where we must be ware too, both in a direct respect, and also in a purchasing respect. It is known that vegetables and fruit deteriorate nutritionally the longer they are stored and so it is important that we purchase as fresh a produce as we can, and likewise use any fresh produce within a short space of time. Where practical, it's a good idea to keep such produce cool, as warmth makes them ripen and deteriorate, far more quickly.

    Sadly there are many pitfalls we must beware of when trying to buy good nutritious food for ourselves these days; whilst a good many purport to be good for us, this is not always the case. Despite their attractive packaging and reassuring words, they cannot always be relied upon as healthy food sources. This is either because such products contain high levels of preservatives, or because they have lost much of their nutritional value during their cooking/production. As already stated, by far the most serious of these two pitfalls lies in respect to the sugars and salts commonly used to preserve such produce. When consumed to excess, both can bring about obesity and high blood pressure conditions. It is also the case that these products (including many children's drinks) often contain chemicals to improve their appearance in respect to colour and their consistency. Fortunately, the food and drinks industries are working hard to address such issues and make such foods more healthy for us.

These days modern farming methods leave a lot to be desired too. In many cases our food is days, weeks or even months old before we get to eat it and so its nutritional content may have diminished quite considerably by the time we get it. This particularly applies to chilled produce from overseas. It is also the case that such produce is often picked before it is ripe (particularly in the case of fruit). This in itself can be a very costly practice nutritionally, since it is known that during the natural ripening process (via interaction with sunlight) vitamin C reaches its peak, and so to short circuit this process can result in the fruits' nutritional benefits being reduced.

It is also the cases that much of the land where our food is grown these days is repeatedly used, which can affect the nutrients contained in these soils. Whereas in the past, land was rotated and allowed to rest, these days land is in constant use. Once depleted of nutrients, the crops grown in such soil sometimes lose much of their goodness. With organically grown crops on the other hand, food grown in such a way is often far more nutritious because the soil used to grow the crops is treated with respect. Instead of chemical fertilizers being used to re-invigorate the land, natural elements such as manure are used to feed and nurture the organisms necessary to process and rejuvenate the soil. The soil is periodically rested too. There is a catch to such production however in that that food produced in this way inevitably costs more, because of the extended time and effort required to produce such food.

At the end of the day you get what you pay for and this is certainly true where nutritious foods are concerned. Sadly whilst fruit and vegetables may look the same, there is no way we can verify their quality other than to trace their production route.

Another area where we must be wary, lies in respect to food/nutritional supplements. Whilst it is true that we can attain many nutrients in a refined form from local health-food shops and on the internet, in the form of vitamin and mineral supplements etc, they are rarely effective as a total substitute for natural forms of nutrition. As their name suggests they are merely supplements to boost our nutrient stocks, rather than act as main nutritional sources.

Being processed chemicals of a highly refined form, they are in effect medicines and should therefore be treated with great respect. Where we do use them, it is important to read the manufacturers instructions printed on any packaging and adhere strictly to the dosage recommendations given. Failure to do so could cause digestive disturbance or have very serious consequence in respect to our health. It should also be noted that whilst supplements of fish oils, evening primrose oil etc are fairly safe, others can interact with prescribed medicines on occasion and so its important to tell or consult a medical practitioner/dietician before starting a course of such medication.

Health restrictions

Whilst we may aim to live a healthy life, much depends upon our physical constitution to a degree and so sadly in some cases we may experienced health problems which require a restricted diet of some kind (i.e. where food intolerances occur). The most common of food intolerances, relating to dairy, nut, or cereal products, can make our lives particularly difficult for example. Fortunately in a good many cases where they do occur at a young age we often tend to grow out of them. Where food intolerances occur at a later age, such problems can often be rectified by avoiding the offending foods for a short time and then introducing them slowly over a matter of weeks or months. Being major nutrient sources it is not wise to avoid dairy produce or cereal foods for too long as this can prove detrimental to our health. Where we do cut out such types of food from our diet we should only do so under medical supervision.

Where negative immune system responses occur (i.e. arthritis, asthma, migraine and M.E.) certain fruits and vegetables can play their part, in either aggravating, or relieving such conditions. In the case of strawberries and red peppers for example, they are known to aggravate conditions such as arthritis because of their high acidity. Many salad vegetables (containing vitamin E which has strong anti-inflammatory properties) are known to be good for such conditions.

Circulatory and digestive disorders are another area where nutritional restrictions can often apply too. Sadly circulatory disorders (i.e. heart conditions etc) are becoming increasingly common as our tendency to exercise diminishes and our preference for processed food increases.

As well as cutting out fatty foods, which will cause us to put on weight and clog up our arteries, it is important to beware of processed/convenience foods, since some of these contain high level of preservatives such as salt, which will increase our blood pressure (certain types of biscuits, i.e. digestives etc can likewise do the same). It is therefore advisable to check food packaging for sodium content and choose those products with the lowest percentages. Fortunately, as I've already indicated, in recent times many convenience food producers have started to make such foods much healthier for us by reformulating these meals in a positive way. They also now put the exact contents of these foods on their packaging with a breakdown of all ingredients too, making it much easier for us to know just what we are eating when we buy such food.

Unfortunately, even though the health food industry is doing its best to make sure our food is healthy these days, in some cases, any failings with food can be down to us, in that we may accidentally let food go out of date, or fail to store it as directed by the producer. Should this happen, we can easily fall victim to digestive tract illnesses such as sickness and diarrhoea. Digestive tract illness may not necessarily be down to something we have eaten however; sometimes we may get sickness or diarrhoea because we have come into contact with a bug of some kind, or our bodies may have decided they do not like something we have ingested. Where digestive disorders occur, they can take many different forms; as well as allergy upsets caused by food intolerances, we may also be prone to stomach ulcers due to stress or through not eating meals on a regular basis too. All of these examples need to be treated in a different ways.

Where we develop sickness/diarrhoea for example, it's important to assess our situation and establish a probable cause, looking at all the food we have eaten over the past few days and where possible, we should check the packaging dates on any cooked meats, tins, mayonnaise/sauces, dairy produce; or any fish produce we have consumed. It might be that we have young children and they might have caught a bug through their social interaction with others and passed something on to us or other close family members We also need to assess where we have been in a social context (i.e. have we been to a social gathering of some kind ? Have we been to a hospital, also whether or not we have bought food from a fast food outlet, or eaten out at a restaurant); all these possibilities need to be assessed thoroughly. As with most other digestive tract illnesses, sickness and diarrhoea can prove very serious if allowed to continue for too long (particularly where small children are concerned) due to the risk of dehydration, which can damage our body's organs. With food poisoning symptoms usually occur from six hours to three days after we have eaten some infected food.

    Having pinpointed when we started to feel ill, and the meals we have eaten just before or around that time, we can then decide upon a course of action. First and foremost (particularly where food poisoning has occurred), we have to deal with pain management and diagnosis.

    Where abdominal pain or sickness is severe, it is best to consult a doctor or medically qualified person as soon as possible. Where symptoms are severe it is unwise to take strong painkillers to mask the pain without medical supervision as this could impair medical assistance, should our situation require medical intervention. Where symptoms are less severe, we can monitor such conditions ourselves and where we feel necessary, book an appointment to see a doctor.

    Often the main problem with sickness/stomach upsets can be keeping food inside ourselves. Where we have a stomach bug, it is often best to avoid meals for a short while until the troublesome bugs have decreased in number, but we should drink plenty of plain fluids. We should then gradually introduce small amounts of food into our system; carefully monitoring our reaction to such foods (such meals should have plain simple constituents however). Foods such as soup toast, bread etc are known to be easier to digest under these circumstances. Light meals such as egg on toast, mashed potato with boiled fish and peas are common examples of such foods, though at the end of the day it comes down to personal choice and what we fancy. Under no circumstances should fried or fatty foods be attempted at such times as these will promote heavy gastric activity, which could upset us again.

      Should we conclude that our illness occurred as a result of food poisoning, we obviously have to act pretty swiftly. Whilst we may not be feeling at our best, it is important to make sure that all foods in our home i.e. in our fridge, cupboards etcetera are fit to be eaten (or if suspected of causing our illness, are disposed of), so as to prevent others in our household from becoming ill, or re-infecting ourselves. Where we suspect that we have become ill as a result of eating out or in a social context, we have a moral obligations to others' particularly the elderly, sick or infirm to let those responsible for providing any suspected food know about our illness so that they can check their food stock, to prevent the risk of others becoming ill. With true food poisoning it's generally the case that we will require some degree of medical assistance to cope with our illness. As part of this process, laboratory tests will usually be authorised by our doctor, so as to determine what bug we have so that it can be treated correctly. Where bugs are of a serious nature, our doctor or the laboratory that conducted the tests will let the authorities know about our illness, particularly so where a doctor medical clinic has had several cases of the same illness made known to them. There will then be an official investigation carried out to try and trace the source of such illness.

      As I've already indicated, digestive disorders can take many different forms; probably the most common forms of such illness being indigestion and stomach ulcers, both need to be taken seriously, as they (like sickness/diarrhoea) can have serious implications. Whilst both conditions can be very uncomfortable, stomach ulcers usually the more serious of these conditions since they can result in major blood loss, sometimes to the point of fatality. Stomach ulcers don't just happen overnight though; they generally develop over several weeks or months. In a good many cases, they are caused by stress, or as a result of missing meals, where our gastric juices burn their way through our stomach lining, though certain types of medication can provoke such conditions on occasion. Fortunately there are several forms of very effective medication which can be used to heal them, but none the less, those suffering such a condition do need to watch their diet to some degree, particularly in respect to fatty food intake, which can in some cases aggravate such conditions. The most important thing with such conditions is that those affected, eat on a regular basis. As well as causing stomach ulcers, it is known that missing meals will seriously aggravate them too.

    By far the most common of gastric conditions is that of reflux (indigestion where the upper part of our stomach becomes sore or inflamed. Such situations can arise for a variety of reasons, but more commonly they are associated with a hiatus hernia, where a small valve at the top of the stomach has become damaged. This erroneously allows digestive acid to rise up into our throat, burning our sensitive throat membranes in the process.

    Whilst indigestion is a very common situation, it can be confused with symptoms of a heart condition because of symptom proximity, though with a heart condition, as well as local pain, pain often occurs in the arms too.

    Fortunately where indigestion is concerned there are a wide range of measures we can take, to both treat, and prevent such occurrences, without the need for surgery or complex medicines. Most pharmacists sell chalk based antacid tablets and protective digestive fluids, which can offer great comfort. Our posture can also make a difference to the severity of symptoms too. It is known that lying flat and bending after meals will aggravate such conditions, as will certain foods (particularly fatty types) and drinks too (drinks such as coffee for example) especially so if they are consumed late at night or just before bedtime.

In all cases where indigestion is concerned, if symptoms occur regularly or on a long-term basis, proper medical investigation may be needed; such conditions should never be taken for granted or ignored. Unfortunately indigestion on a regular basis, if left untreated, could cause permanent damage to the lining of our throat. It is therefore, as I've indicated, important to get such symptoms medically checked out.

There are also several other digestive disorders which can cause us problems too; irritable bowel syndrome and diverticulitis are probably the most common of these. With irritable bowel syndrome, a whole host of inexplicable reasons can trigger such conditions, i.e. an allergy, stress etc; it can therefore be very difficult to pin down an exact cause to this illness. One of the best ways to manage this condition is to keep a food and general diary, and to refer to your diary when symptoms occur. This can often help to identify foods or situations which trigger such conditions.

In the cased of diverticulitis, where the lower stomach develops small bulging sacs; this is a situation which seems to occur more frequently in older people (from middle age onwards). These bulging sacs can sometimes trap food and become infected, leading to great pain and possible complications. In respect to the treatment for diverticulitis; it is known that consuming too much rough fibre, nuts, cereal bran etc can aggravate the condition, therefore softer sources of fibre should be consumed instead. It is particularly important to takes such steps during episodes of illness. It is also a bad idea to consume too many stodgy foods on a regular basis too, since such foods can aggravate the condition.

One of the most serious digestive conditions, comes in the form of diabetes. If left untreated or unmanaged, diabetes can cause blindness, nervous collapse, hear attacks, strokes, loss of limbs and a whole host of other very serious life threatening conditions. Diabetes must therefore always be taken seriously should it be discovered in someone.

Sadly this particularly nasty illness is becoming increasingly common these days thanks in part to our over-consumption of sweet and heavily processed foods. (Genetic pre-disposition can and does also play a part in illness susceptibility too of course.)

There are basically two forms of diabetes; Type 1 and type 2. Whilst both are very serious, type 1 is far more so. That s because with this version of the illness, an essential chemical (insulin) which helps us is turn glucose sugar into energy does not get produced by the pancreas as it should do. Because of this, sufferers of this condition can be virtually poisoned by an overload of unusable energy. In the case of type 1 diabetes, sufferers of this type, generally have to inject themselves regularly with insulin in order to overcome this situation, in order to make their bodies work as they should. With type two diabetes (where insulin function does not work very well), dietary management can often be enough to keep the condition in check, though medical monitoring is still required. The most alarming thing about this condition however can be its ability to remain unnoticed until symptoms are well advanced.

Fortunately the medical profession is always on the lookout for this nasty illness and it is often during routine tests that the condition is picked up. In the case of both types of diabetes, a radical change in diet will be required to keep the condition in check. There are a whole host of foods which should be avoided.

The most important foods to avoid when suffering diabetes are as follows: i.e. sugary sweets, cakes and pastry, fatty meats, sweetened fruit drinks; full fat milk/dairy produce, dried fruits such as apricots, dates raisins etc, white bread, chips and other fried foods. Not only do these foods contain too much sugar for diabetics to handle, they can also bring about serious weight gain which can also cause problems in respect to the condition. Low fat dairy produce and some types of fruit can be beneficial under supervision. It is also important to ensure that an adequate amount of fluids are consumed too, as dehydration is always a risk in respect to diabetes.

Whilst it is a very complex and serious condition, with careful dietary management and medical supervision it is possible to live a normal life even with this condition, by sticking to plain and simple foods, and by taking regular exercise. It is now believed that if those with type 2 diabetes abstain from problem foods at an early stage of the illness, it can sometimes be possible to overcome this disease, though research is still going on into this possibility.

Women's health

As I've already indicated, it's especially important that the metabolic needs of women are taken into account where diets are concerned (from puberty, right through to old age). Where young girls are concerned, it is particularly important that they get a good nutritional start in life. All through their lives women require good nutrition. Probably the most important elements they require are iron, calcium and B group vitamins. If women are to stay healthy for the duration of their lives, they must take in these essential nutrients on a regular basis (particularly calcium, in order to ward off the risk of osteoporosis). Fortunately these essential nutrients can all be readily obtained from meat and dairy produce (though such foods are not favoured by everyone. Where people chose a vegetarian lifestyle, they will probably be able to get sufficient B group vitamins from fruit, nuts and vegetables (much depends upon the quality of those vegetables etc). In all cases where a vegetarian diet is undertaken careful supervision and monitoring by a qualified medical practitioner will be required to ensure that no serious nutritional deficiencies occur.

In some cases additional supplementation will be required; this particularly applies during later years when our bodies function less efficiently. From puberty onwards, women are also subject to certain metabolic conditions too i.e. P.M.S, the menopause, osteoporosis etc, all of these situations can be positively influenced by suitable dietary management. It is known that the symptoms of P.M.S can be greatly reduced by taking regular exercise, eating small meals on a regular basis (particularly carbohydrates such as biscuits etc) and by taking B group supplements where necessary (particularly B6). It is also wise to avoid acidic foods, white bread and sugar, as these are known to aggravate symptoms.

During later life, a woman's metabolism changes very dramatically as she reaches and passes through the menopause. Not only can such experiences be physically uncomfortable, they can also have major mental repercussions too as her treasured fertility ebbs away. Fortunately theses days the process can be managed very effectively, thanks to modern medicines. It is however, still up to those affected to adjust and cope with this major transitional period in their lives and any long-term repercussions that may present themselves. As I've already indicated, our diet can make a great difference in respect to the severity of symptoms. One major factor which can be of benefit, both during the changes and after, can be regular exercise. Not only will this help to keep our body tissue in shape, but it is known that the adrenal glands take over female hormone management once the menopause has occurred, and so by exercising we can ensure that such hormones are distributed around the body on a regular basis.

Dieting

Dieting can take many different forms and for a very wide range of reasons. In some cases we may be concerned about our physical profile. In other cases we may have experienced bad health as a result of our being overweight, or been advised by our doctor to lose some weight. Regardless of circumstances, in all cases, a substantial degree of willpower will be required on our part.

Like all things, there are ways to make such tasks easier. Having the support of others can make a great difference for example. It can often be a good idea to enrol in a slimming group. That way we can share the experiences and triumphs of others, which will hopefully spur us on to achieve our own goals. Likewise when we are finding our task difficult, others within such groups can often provide valuable support and encouragement.

Whilst it is harder to lose weight and easy to get dispirited when attempting weight loss on our own, much depends upon our approach to our task, as to whether we will be successful or not. In both approaches, a standard set of rules apply. Firstly our choice of diet must be palatable to us. All too often people fail when trying to lose weight simply because they have been over zealous, either in respect to their choice of restricted foods, or in some cases the amount of physical food they allow themselves.

To restrict our diet in respect to food range can often be a recipe for disaster in that we often find ourselves craving those foods we have chosen to deny ourselves and so unless we are very strong willed, we can often be tempted to give in to temptation; this will obviously undermine our efforts. The best policy is therefore to restrict the physical amount of fattening foods we consume rather than cut them out completely. In many cases we can fill our plate with healthier alternatives such as salad vegetables, lettuce, cabbage etc. Instead of having four potatoes just have one, or possibly two, (taking care to reduce the size of garnishes too, i.e. salad creams mayonnaise etc). We should also pay attention to the types of food and the way that food is prepared/cooked. Where possible, meats should be grilled, and drained of residual fat by way of kitchen role (as applies to chips too).

It is also the case that restrictive and starvation diets can pose a serious health risk, in that we may be depriving ourselves of essential nutrients, or in some cases where one particular food is recommended, that food could poison us (i.e. through an overload of vitamin A found in vegetables, particularly carrots for example. Mono-food diets should therefore be avoided unless specifically recommended by a qualified medical practitioner and for sound medical reasons.

The greatest weapon in respect to losing weight however can be physical exercise. Rather than just restricting the food we eat, the magic ingredient in respect to losing weight is undoubtedly exercise undertaken together with our diet. Without a suitable exercise regime we are far less likely to lose significant amounts of weight. Where we do decide to incorporate an exercise routine into our slimming regime, it's important to take things steady to start off with, especially so where we're not used to taking exercise, as it is all too easy to pull muscles, tendons etc, where our muscle tone is poor. Ideally it is best to participate in a controlled exercise class, as this should ensure we get adequate supervision in respect to warm up/warm down routines, at a pace we can cope with.

It is true that slimming pills etc exist, but these mainly work by promoting the expulsion of fluids from our bodies (diuretics). Sadly such methods are seldom effective long-term, since any fluids lost will accumulate once again when such medication ceases. It is also the case that we risk dehydration by using such methods and run the risk of liver/kidney damage in some cases (where such methods are used without medical supervision).

Probably the most effective slimming method requires a three pronged attack, as well as exercise, and dietary self-discipline, a course of massage sessions can be a great help too, in that the masseur will be able to break down those areas of static body fat so that they can be voided from our systems. Certain aromatherapy oils can be very effective in this (i.e. cypress and juniper for example).

Where we do try to lose weight, we should be prepared for a long haul in most cases. Whilst it is true that some people can shed pounds in a very short time, in a good many cases they tend to put their weight back on just as quickly. This is often because they have taken a dietary shortcut of the type I've just mentioned (through using pills or a starvation diet).

Losing weight can also be something of a nutritional learning experience too. Because we are all individuals, certain foods can affect us more than others in respect to putting on weight. In some cases potatoes will cause people to put on weight, in others pasta or other foods can affect us. Losing weight therefore largely comes down to personal experience, self-discipline and vigilance (by way of regular weight monitoring) on our part. Certain medical procedures are also favoured by some, but such procedures can prove very disruptive to our lives and so careful consideration needs to be given to the repercussions of such a step, along with a full medical consultation, before we physically undertake any such procedures.

STRESS

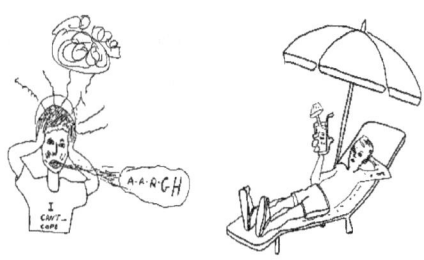

Like it or not we are all subject to the stresses of life (good and bad), just as we have been all through history. Stresses are not always bad for us however; in many cases stresses can have a positive, beneficial effect upon us too. Stresses can for example provide us with an incentive to take action in some way when we are under some kind of threat; they generate mental and physical movement in one form or another.

Without stress we wouldn't be able to function. Feeding ourselves is a prime example. Whilst it is true that most of our bodily functions, i.e. breathing, the digestion of food etc, occur automatically, we still have to consciously find and eat food to sustain ourselves. It is the stress of hunger which forces us to act, since we know, either as a result of bodily pain, or experience, that we must find food to sustain ourselves (a stress which is at the very root of our existence). Stresses are therefore an essential aspect of our lives.

We also have other needs (on an emotional level), which relate to stress as well, companionship, and stimulation, by way of challenges for example (i.e. sporting pursuits and hobbies etc). Whilst our circumstances can vary greatly in respect to companionship (i.e. we get lonely without friends/partners, or alternatively dislike crowds/social events) all of us have a competitive hunting instinct buried within us to some degree. The focus of our challenges and companionship needs can and does vary greatly from individual to individual. Some of us are avid collectors, others have strong sporting desires, either as competitors or as spectators; life would be pretty dull without such objectives. Regardless of their form, all of these stresses serve a positive purpose for our own good.

There are also many negatives associated with stress too of course. In some cases stresses can bring about metabolic changes within us, which can in some cases prove harmful to us; i.e. they can increase our blood pressure, which can make us susceptible to heart attacks, strokes etc. Stress can equally be responsible for a wide range of mental disorders too, including depression, temper tantrums and forgetfulness, all of which are clearly detrimental to our wellbeing. Where stresses are concerned, we therefore have to manage our lives and experiences effectively if we are to avoid such conditions.

Stress management

Stress management can take many different forms and apply in many contexts. In some cases stress management involves preventative measures, i.e. insurances etc, in other cases stress management involves problem solving techniques. In other cases where stresses are unavoidable, stress management applies in a direct sense through coping strategies etc.
    Of the situations which are known to cause us stress, bereavement, job loss, holidays, relationship breakdowns, looking after others who are ill, moving house and mechanical failure are amongst the worst situations we have to deal with. How we react under these circumstances can make a considerable difference in respect to our well-being; much depends upon our personality to a degree. Some of us are happy go lucky people who take all things in our stride, whilst others tend to get very angry when stressed, or else worry quite unnecessarily over the most trivial of situations; worrying won't change a situation however. In most cases, where we encounter stress, we need to take direct action of some kind (a typical example of this being where we are ill). If we are not careful we can worry ourselves to a point of great distress, when there is really no need. By having the courage to visit our doctor, we can often have our minds put our mind at rest; or if something is wrong, we can have some confidence that the issue will be sorted out in most cases. Under these circumstances it is generally the case the longer we leave our problems the worse they will get. This applies to a great many situations of course. Getting angry can likewise be just as counterproductive, particularly where machinery is involved.

Whilst it is only too easy to get frustrated with machinery when it fails to respond to our commands, under these circumstances, we often have no option but to accept our situation and deal with it objectively. Either the machinery is broken, or we need to learn how to operate it correctly. There's no point in getting angry with a piece of machinery since it is in no position to respond. If we are violent with machinery we are merely likely to break it and so we will be put to more expense in respect to having to buy a new machine, or in getting our original one repaired.

Sadly in this day and age we are becoming evermore dependent upon such machinery and fast losing control of our lives as a result. Whereas in the past we could act directly to do something, now in most cases we are reliant upon some type of machinery, either in the context of a labour saving device, or as a storage facility. Such machinery tends to increases our stress loading tremendously, not only in respect to usage problems but also in respect to cost. It is far too late to turn the clock back however, we must therefore accept the role mechanical and electronic devices now play in our lives and use them accordingly. In many cases this can be easier said than done (particularly with electronic gadgetry). None the less we have to adapt to such changes and learn to cope with the stresses which such machinery may at times cause us (and that modern life in general can cause us too).

When we encounter stressful situations, we need to establish if and how we can change them to our advantage. If we can't change them, we must accept them and make ourselves as comfortable with our new circumstances as we can (relationship breakdowns etc). Whilst this is not an ideal situation, there are many different ways we can minimise/counteract the effect such stressful experiences will have upon us, particularly when our stresses involve others, i.e. where close friends, relatives etc are in some kind of trouble for example. When it comes to stress management, all our options will require a great deal of self-discipline and reasoning on our part.

One obvious way we can protect ourselves from stress lies in respect to insurances for example. Where things are going well it's all too easy to assume they will continue that way; sadly things can all too easily go wrong for us as we all know. If we own a car, we may have an accident; if we own a house it could catch fire; if we are self-employed we could fall ill etc. Whilst none of these situations are pleasant to think about, all would have a terrible impact upon us and our lives should they occur. It is therefore essential that we have contingency plans, both to give ourselves peace of mind so that we don't need to worry about such situations, and more importantly, physical protection, so that we don't end up without a car, homeless etc. Fortunately there are a great many insurance providers around us. Although we may resent paying out premiums for such insurances, it's important to realise that proportionally such premiums are often minimal in respect to any payouts we may require (i.e. house insurance) and the security such policies give us.

In all areas of our life, there is one element which can aid us tremendously, that being communication, either in respect to negotiating difficult situations, or more importantly, in sharing our feelings when we are greatly stressed. Through communication we can often secure the empathy/wisdom of others, both of which can help us to get over any difficult times and situations. Often while we're talking to others we come up with solutions to problems of our own accord, without the need of other people's wisdom (that is the purpose of counselling). If on the other hand we keep our stresses bottled up inside ourselves, this can easily lead to ill health (both, physical and mental) or relationship breakdown.

It is also essential that we listen to the needs/requirements of others too (especially where family relationships are concerned, i.e. partners, children etc).

Stress relief

Sadly stressful problems are all around us, we encounter them on a regular basis, on both a personal, and a professional level and so we have no option but to accept and deal with them as best we can. Regardless of the cause or circumstances for life's pressures/stresses, they should all be handled in the same way, by way of the following steps – firstly when under stress, we need to evaluate the circumstances of our stress in an objective, unbiased way, putting our own instinctive preferences for action to one side, and look at our situation from all sides/angles. This is particularly important where our situation involves others, in that by doing so, we can often empathise with our opposite number (make compromises where necessary) and so avoid costly arguments, thus ensuring the valuable co-operation of those around us. It is essential that we evaluate all situations of course; no matter whether we are trying to repair a broken item, use complex machinery or plan a career etc. In all cases we need to look at our options seriously and in detail before we act.

Sadly the old maxim act in haste repent at leisure is all too true. The time we have for evaluation can often be limited, but in all situations, some degree of evaluation is necessary. Most importantly, we need to consider the negative aspects of any courses of action we may be planning to take (should there be any), prior to taking any action; not in the context of aborting a planned course of action, but so that we are prepared as to how to deal with a negative outcome of our actions.

Finally we need to decide upon and take some form of action; where possible making sure we can reverse our decision (or at least lessen the impact of our decision, if we have acted in error). In life, it's all too easy to make wrong decisions, but awfully hard to put things right, i.e. disagreements with employers, family members, etc. The use of computerised equipment and digital phones illustrates this only too clearly. When using such equipment i.e. computers, phones etc, it is all too easy to press the wrong button or chose the wrong option, with disastrous consequences.

All too often we act in desperation and we choose the most straightforward option at the time, or else we tend to wrestle with our problems head on until we are weary and too tired to resolve them. Where problems/difficult situations are concerned however, it is often best to step back from them and view them from a distance, at our leisure. Whilst this is not always possible, it is generally the case that the most successful problem resolutions do come about in this way. That is why businessmen get more work done during social occasions, when they are more relaxed. Diversions undoubtedly serve a very beneficial purpose (provided we are strict with ourselves and don't just use such occasions to avoid our problems). On a domestic level, word-search puzzles, crossword/jigsaw puzzles etc serve a very similar purpose, as of course do walks in the country, along the beach etc. Indeed relaxation and diversions are by far the greatest weapons we have against life's stresses and so where possible we should use them to our full advantage.

Many "alternative" therapies are known to be very effective at relieving stress too (i.e. massage, reflexology, visualisation, meditation therapy etc). As well as providing treatment for stress conditions, some "alternative" therapies and practices can actually protect us again stress, yoga and meditation being prime examples (see pages 60 – 62 and 141 - 143). There are also other measures we can take to relax us by way of our environment too. Soft coloured decor/house furnishings for example, cuddly toys, pictures, certain types of music etc can all help us to stay calm and relaxed if we are willing to use them. Pets can likewise help us in our battle against stress too.

Self belief

In terms of stress, self-belief can be a vital element in our coping strategy; exams, job interviews etcetera are a prime example. If we are less than confident in respect to any tasks we undertake, we are likely to become tired or highly stressed as a result of our anxiety, both are likely to hamper our task. Where exam situations are concerned, it is important to learn as much about our subject as we can, well in advance of any exams.

Ideally it's advisable to study very hard during the early part of a course, so that we are reasonably confident in respect to our knowledge of the subject or subjects we are to be tested on. By doing this we will hopefully feel more relaxed around the time running up to the exam. We then just have to undertake detailed revision of our subject or subjects and brush up on any areas where we feel less confident. This very much depends upon our degree of willpower, memory capability and circumstances to a degree however, but as I've already indicated, to try and learn everything at the last minute, or during the final months of a course can be a recipe for disaster. In some cases our minds can become overloaded by last minute studying and so we are unable to think clearly. Making us become muddle headed and anxious about the task which lies ahead of us. Much depends upon our long-term memory to a degree, for studying well in advance does not suit everyone. Some people actually benefit from last minute cramming where their long-term memory is not very good. We are all different in this respect and so it is down to how well we know ourselves at the end of the day.

During the final hours before an exam, it is sometimes a good idea to take some time out for ourselves, by doing something we enjoy, by going shopping, pursuing a favourite hobby etc; something which will take our mind off the task which lies ahead of us so that we don't start to worry. As I've already indicated however, with tests and exams, this course of action is not always appropriate, as those with a poor long-term memory can sometimes benefit from last minute cramming and focussing on the exam or exams ahead of them.

Where we do become anxious over exams and tests, this often makes concentration very difficult. This can be clearly seen where we are endeavouring to pass our driving test for example. In most cases we will have mastered the controls of a vehicle to the point where our instructor is sure we can pass, but at the end of the day, it's often how we feel in an emotional context that will determine our fate. The same applies in the case of job interviews too. When faced with such situations, familiarity of our subject and practical knowledge of job requirements/company policy etc can be crucial, but likewise so can our attitude as well. A great many people without suitable qualifications have bluffed their way through interviews and landed a top job, even though they were under qualified. Likewise a great many highly qualified persons have failed at interviews simply because they were anxious and gave the impression they would prove incompetent if given the job.

Our subconscious thought processes can in some cases determine our general luck in life too; as such examples prove only too clearly (see also self hypnosis pages 138 - 141).

Whilst being confident can clearly be an asset in life, being overconfident can often prove to be detrimental, either because we come unstuck and make mistakes or do damage (as applies to some drivers), or because others feel threatened by our manner, or resent such confidence, seeing it as arrogance. There can be no doubt however that those with genuine confidence suffer far less in terms of stress than those who are less than confident.

Whilst unfamiliarity should rightly provoke apprehension in terms of safety, no one should ever feel intimidated by new experiences as there are always opportunities available for us to learn how to deal with such situations. In most cases it is just a question of consulting someone, openly and calmly who is familiar with the situation we are unsure as to how to deal with, or conducting a little research on our part, via books the internet etc; or where immediate situations occur, taking things cautiously, thinking through the results of any actions we may be tempted to take, before we choose or chose not to act on a situation we are confronted with.

Social interaction

The way in which we deal with our family and others can also make a tremendous difference to our lives, both on a positive note (in the form of support and mutual co-operation), or on a negative note, in respect to arguments/disagreements. Whilst the former can most definitely work to our advantage, the reverse is certainly the case where arguments and ill feeling arise.

Where social interactive stresses are concerned, it is generally a good idea for us to do as much for ourselves as we can whilst running our lives. Relying upon others to do things for us is a well-proven emotional minefield. People are often willing to offer their help, but all too often they get side-tracked by their own direct priorities and so our particular task can sometimes get forgotten or delayed. Sadly these situations can and frequently do cause great friction within relationships. Where we ask for the help of others, we should therefore be prepared for some degree of disappointment. As such events prove, interacting with others can be extremely stressful at times.

On occasion we do need to assert our authority and make our feelings known in a forceful manner if we are to get our needs/wishes fulfilled; that said however, to generate, or be involved in ill feeling, is most definitely bad for us. Sadly many people have suffered serious health problems (or in some cases died), as a result of an argument, over something very trivial. We must therefore evaluate such occasions very carefully.

Where disagreements are concerned, it is only too easy to stick to our guns when we believe we are right, often to the point of a serious argument (road rage being a prime example), or alternatively, take criticism to heart, both threaten our health to a degree; even if we win an argument, we are still likely to suffer as a result of ill feeling. Where possible it is often best to give in to an argument graciously (provided it's not too costly for us), or at least negotiate a suitable compromise if there is one.

Not only is losing our temper bad for us healthwise, losing our temper is also bad for us in relationship terms where we are interacting with others too, in that it never pays to fall out with people in case we need their help or co-operation in the future. (There can be nothing more humiliating than having to ask for help from someone we have fallen out with.) Whilst it is not always practical to do so, where possible it is generally a good idea to count to ten psychologically under our breath when we are angry with someone, or leave an area of great stress or confrontation, until we are calm enough to deal constructively with a difficult situation or conversation.

The problems of others, can bring us great stress if we're not careful too. Where the problems of others are concerned we often have little or no control over events; it is important that we realise and accept this. It is true that we can give advice, but all too often, others choose to ignore such advice and so we can be left feeling very frustrated on occasion. Under these circumstances, we should be content in the fact that we have tried to help those concerned and accept that at the end of the day there's little more we can do, other than to support them should their condition or situation worsen.

It is all too easy lying awake at night worrying about either our own, or other people's problems; by doing so we won't solve other people's problems. In most cases worrying will just make us ill or extremely tired, which will put us at risk of emotional or physical harm (where we are operating dangerous machinery or driving for example).

In some cases, stresses can put considerable strain upon relationships too, by making us tired, depressed, or more commonly irritable. Stress can also affect our sex lives as well, making us sexually impotent in some cases. Whilst such a situation will be distressing for both partners, fortunately in a good many cases such problems can often be resolved by simply examining our stress loading. It may be that our work situation is making us too tired, we may be worried by previous experiences, our health etc. In most cases it's just a case of locating the cause of our stress, and regaining our sexual confidence. Probably the best way to do so is to take subsequent sexual encounters slowly for a while, making the most of foreplay techniques such as mutual massage etc; by doing so, we will become far more relaxed in respect to our task, and hopefully become more successful in our endeavours. Should we encounter long-term issues, it is often wise to get ourselves medically checked out so that serious medical conditions can be ruled out.

Where we have children they can likewise be a big worry for us too, not just in respect to their actions but also in respect to their general welfare at the hands of others (bullies etc). Although we may not be able to give them round the clock protection in a physical sense, we do have a powerful weapon at our disposal in respect to communication. Whilst parenting styles vary greatly, it has been found that the best friend approach is generally more effective than the dominant style of parenting, in that children often respect their parents far more in the long-term. They are more ready to accept a parents' guidance too, whereas children of dominant parents may be more rebellious. Much depends upon the children concerned in this respect, but it is a fact that all children are vulnerable and like to experiment. They likewise like to make decisions for themselves (good and bad). It is therefore far better that children can share their plans and experiences with their parents without fear of chastisement. If something bad happens to them, parents are likely to know soon after an incident and can take immediate action, whereas children who fear being told off, will keep any bad experiences quiet. The best friend style of parenting has proven long-term relationship benefits too of course.

Where children are very young, communication is difficult and so we do need to be ever vigilant in respect to their welfare. There are things we can do though, in respect to window locks, protective barriers, and the keeping of medicines, household chemicals, high up out of their reach. All these courses of action will go some way to giving us peace of mind.

Time-pressures

No matter whether it, is our partner, children, friends, or relatives, the allocation of our time is an issue which is bound to leave us feeling extremely stressed on occasion. For many of us, our lives are mapped out for us from day one.

    Regardless of what we may want to do in our early years, we are dependent upon our parents and so by and large we have to live by their rules. Besides them setting our mealtimes/bedtimes etc, we are also required to attend school, which takes up a major part of our time. Whilst we may wish for the opportunity to play our computer games etc, we have to live according to the timeslots dictated by others.

    As we reach adulthood time pressures increase radically, in that our need for finance means we have to get a job, and work according to the timeslots/constraints allocated by others (where we are employed to make deliveries being a prime example). We are also likely to be romantically involved with someone in a good many cases, which will also increase time pressures put upon us, as we try to accommodate their needs.

    Where we have a family, time pressures can at times seem unbearable as everyone maps out our day. Children want our attention, to be taken to school, or out to see friends; our partner often wants us to do jobs around the home, our employer wanting us to work the maximum number of hours, often we have financial deadlines to meet in the form of bills etc. Sadly few of us can escape such pressures, but what we can do is to manage these situations as I've already indicated through negotiation, so that we have relative harmony around us. The principle rule where time is concerned is that of prioritisation, whereby we assess and aim to meet our most pressing time commitments, according to their impact upon us should we fail to meet each particular deadline. The same applies in respect to monetary issues too.

Financial pressures

No matter who we are, we all need money to pay bills, leisure commitments etc. Much depends upon our circumstances and personalities to a degree, but in all cases, regardless of income, we need to manage our finances according to our income if we are to avoid the stresses financial commitments can bring.
    We need to eat, we need to have a roof over our head; these are two undisputable commitments. When we consider our finances these two priorities therefore have to come first and foremost, closely followed by clothing and companionship. In most cases money has to be earned and so we have to persuade others to employ us in one context or another (which is not always easy). Having earned our money, we then have to divide our income according to our expenses. If we are lucky we will have some left over to treat ourselves, or be able to save some for future use (much depends upon our range of professional skills in this respect).
    Probably the greatest cause of stress in monetary terms lies in respect to debt. Sadly it is only too easy to run up debt, either because we lack willpower where expenditure management is concerned, or more commonly, because of misplaced optimism in respect to our earnings potential. Whilst it is relatively easy to find others who are willing to lend us money, that money still has to be paid back at some point.
    Although we may be confident when we borrow money, our circumstances can easily change; either we lose our job for some reason, or we become ill and cannot work, both are disastrous when we have borrowed a large sum of money. Unfortunately these situations occur very often, particularly in respect to house purchases where we take out a mortgage (undoubtedly our largest purchase). When things go wrong for us, they often do so in a big way. We must therefore take this into account when we take on a mortgage. As with any loan we must be realistic about our income

rather than optimistic, and never borrow more than we can comfortably afford to pay back.

Where we do take out a loan and get into difficulties it is important that we let our financiers know at the earliest opportunity, it is often possible to have repayments re-scheduled to take our changed circumstances into account, though this does very much depend upon the goodwill of the lender. The same applies in the case of utilities too (gas electricity, telephone companies etc). What we must never do is to ignore a financial problem, no matter how big that problem may seem. The sooner we deal with such problems the sooner they can be resolved. Where we do get our finances in a mess, it can often be a good idea to talk to the Citizens Advice Bureau as they have specialist advisers who can assess our situation objectively; they will know the most effective way to resolve our problems.

As with most other stresses, communication is the key. Through communication we can usually come to some sort of repayment compromise with our lender.

Transport stresses

Transport stresses are a particularly common problem these days, due in part to our hectic schedules but also in respect to the machinery we now rely upon to get us about. Whereas we used to be in direct control of our mobility, by walking, (or in some cases by way of a horse) we are now either dependent upon some form of machinery, i.e. the motorcar/motorcycle or an operator/transport service, i.e. a bus/coach or train service. All can prove a great source for frustration in their own way. Probably the most common source of frustration in this respect relates to car journeys, though bus and train journeys are not far behind; all pose distinctly different but very powerful stresses in their own way. Where we rely upon a bus, train or aeroplane for example, we have to fit in with a company's schedules, which all too frequently fail to match reality, making us late for important business meetings etc on occasion.

    In some cases as individuals we can find the prospect of surrendering control to others, (i.e. nominated drivers/pilots) an unacceptable situation because of our losing direct control. Such circumstances are frequently at the route of stress disorders such as a fear of flying for example. For some, such conditions can be extremely disruptive in respect to holidays, business commitments etc. Fortunately in the case of flying, fears there are a great many ways to resolve such situations, though each require a degree of courage/determination. Besides a degree of counselling, hypnosis can also be a great help (see pages 68-78). Many airlines also run fear of flying courses too whereby they take nervous fliers for short flights with trained psychologists/cabin staff on board to help those with such fears to conquer them. These courses can be most effective, though at the end of the day probably the greatest incentive comes from the freedom which conquering such fears can give us (particularly where we are desperate to see loved ones/family who have moved overseas for example).

People also have fears in respect to busses and trains too but these are often easier to control. More often than not we are able to drive to our destinations instead. Driving in itself can be extremely stressful on today's overcrowded roads however. In a good many cases stresses occur, as a result of either ourselves, or others failing to allow enough time for our/their journeys, though it is also the case (particularly where motorways are concerned) that roadworks can likewise cause us considerable problems on occasion. Besides obviously allowing ourselves more time for our journeys, a little research is often called for where we are unfamiliar with our route, either in respect to getting lost, or in respect to any roadworks along our preferred route.

There are also a whole host of other stresses associated to motor vehicles too of course both in respect to purchase/maintenance costs and also the acquisition of a licence (see self belief, pages 126 - 129). Where vehicle purchases are concerned, a great deal depends upon our finances, as with most purchases. Whilst it is best to spend as much as we can afford to when buying a car, purchasing an older/cheaper car needn't necessarily put us at a disadvantage, much depends upon how the vehicle has been driven and maintained prior to our purchase. Regardless of circumstances, where stress is concerned, it certainly pays dividends to have our car checked over at regular intervals by a competent/qualified mechanic. Whilst this may prove rather costly in financial terms, failure to do so can have far greater costs in emotional terms should our vehicle break down through lack of maintenance.

SELF HYPNOSIS

As the preceding pages illustrate (see self-belief pages 129 - 129), self-belief is essential if we are to prosper in today's world. Believing in ourselves can be a very difficult in some cases however. Probably the most successful method to gain self-belief (besides positive experience), lies in respect to some degree of hypnosis, either in the form of professional assistance (see hypnotherapy section pages 68-78), or possibly through self-hypnosis (see pages 138 -141).

Whilst both procedures of hypnosis can be equally successful, self-hypnosis does require greater self-discipline if such a technique is to be successful. Whereas with managed hypnosis, a professional therapist is on hand to guide us in the direction we wish to go in; with self-hypnosis, it is up to us and us alone to direct our path to success.

As I've already indicated (see hypnotherapy section), the process of hypnosis is a very simple one, one where we aim to use an extremely relaxed state of mind to adjust our behaviour. Although we may not realise it, we pass through the hypnotic state at least twice a day, when we're waking up in the morning, and most importantly, when we're going off to sleep at night. In many cases we unwittingly harness the power of hypnosis with our partners by way of the pillow-talk scenario, when we want something from them, or for them to do something for us. Naturally we try to pick the most appropriate time when they are relaxed, are off their guard and most amenable to our requests. Where we live alone such times (i.e. bedtimes) are often best for us to practice self-hypnosis too, especially so where we are intending to go to sleep, as this will allow our thoughts to crystallise within our subconscious whilst we are sleeping (as can happen where our last thoughts of the day turn into dreams for example).

Self hypnosis, can like general supervised hypnosis, be applied in a great many contexts, either physically, to help us amend our behaviour in some way, i.e. in respect to our wishing to stop smoking, chewing our nails etc, or in a mental context, where we are seeking more confidence etc. In all cases, the key thing is to be clearly focussed as to what we want to achieve before we start; also where psychological changes are required, the implications in respect to our existing relationships, work situation etc, as once we are successful, our perspective on many aspects of our life will undoubtedly change. Sadly if we're not careful, some behavioural changes can cause frictions within relationships; i.e. where we have a partner and we suddenly become more assertive, or we resent the fact that they still smoke etc. When addressing any imperfections we have, we must therefore be very careful and monitor our post hypnotic behaviour very closely; where necessary making adjustments to suit our requirements or circumstances.

  As regards the procedures for self-hypnosis they are relatively simple. First and foremost we need to ensure we have complete privacy from the outside world when trying self-hypnosis. For such a technique to be successful it is essential to choose a time and environment where we can relax completely. That means disconnecting the phone/switching off our mobile etc, choosing a time when we're not likely to be disturbed by others and have no pressing engagements or deadlines to meet. Having found such a window of opportunity, we then have to apply great willpower and focus determinedly upon our chosen goal. Having made ourselves physically relaxed, by taking off our shoes and seated ourselves in a comfortable chair (or ideally retired to the comfort of our bed); it is then a question of finding a physical object to focus upon. This might be a doorknob, a picture, even a crack in the ceiling; the object of our focus doesn't really matter, the main thing is that we can focus our thoughts.

Having found an object to physically focus on we should then stare at that object until we start to feel our eyes getting tired and then slowly close our eyes (whilst continuing to focus upon that object we have chosen to focus on). It can then be a good idea to acknowledge how comfortable we feel and acknowledge how it feels to have all our organs in a relaxed state; to mentally acknowledge that our arms, legs etc are relaxed, to focus on each organ and acknowledge that they are relaxed, from our head and shoulders, right down to our fingers and toes. Most importantly it's important to regulate one's breathing, to acknowledge each breath we draw, and which we allow to leave our body. As we breath out it can also be helpful to whisper the word relax in time with our slow exhaled breath.

Once we are sure we are relaxed we can then concentrate wholly upon those aspects we wish to change. Where we feel it necessary, we can tell ourselves physically that we can for example stop smoking, that we can gain more confidence etc. By adopting such techniques on a regular basis (the number of times vary from person to person), any errant behaviour can be corrected. Likewise when we go to sleep, if we focus upon our goals in a positive mental way they will become that much easier to achieve. With hypnosis belief is everything. If we believe we can, then we can, often achieve our goals.

MEDITATION

Whilst many of the therapies in this book will help with stress, it should be noted that undoubtedly one of the most successful methods of coping with and preventing stress can be to use meditation techniques on a regular basis. It may suit some people to meditate first thing in the morning (before they start their busy day) or during a busy day or last thing at night. Whichever method of meditating is chosen this therapy will undoubtedly be of considerable benefit to the person undertaking such a routine.

Being very similar to self-hypnosis, the steps required to attain a state of meditation are very similar i.e. having found such a window of opportunity you then have to apply great willpower, and focus determinedly upon shutting out the world around you, whilst at the same time focussing inwardly upon yourself. Having made ourselves physically relaxed, by taking off your shoes and seating yourself comfortably in a chair or on the ground or floor, it is then a question of finding a physical object to focus upon. Some people chose to imagine themselves a coloured pyramid or some kind of bubble and this helps to separate us from our physical surroundings. The imagined setting is not so important so much as the process of separating ourselves from direct reality which matters during the induction process. Some people chose to have calming soothing music playing in the background at such times. Other people deem suitable lighting conditions as a priority, choosing to draw the curtains to shut out the light, or if the room is dark, they may dim the lights so that they are soft, or else will light candles with essential oils or perfumes. Others will have a chanting procedure or a guiding narrative recording which they might use. There are a whole range of procedures people will undertake prior to entering meditation.

Having made ourselves comfortable; as with the process of hypnosis, it can then be a good idea to acknowledge how comfortable we feel, and to acknowledge how it feels to have all our organs in a relaxed state; to mentally acknowledge that our arms, legs etc are relaxed, to focus on each organ and acknowledge that they are relaxed, from our head and shoulders, right down to our fingers and toes. Most importantly, it's important to regulate one's breathing, to acknowledge each breath we draw and each breath we allow to leave our body. As we breath out, it can also be helpful to whisper the word relax in time with our slow exhaled breath. We should also try to hold our breath in for a few seconds, and then breathe out in a slow controlled way, pausing slightly, before we draw more breath into our bodies. Some people physically count as they are going through this routine.

Whilst we may be shutting down our consciousness; that does not physically mean going to sleep but instead we should stay in a calm and focussed state of mind. We should then slowly channel our thoughts and focus on something (maybe a beautiful flower or an imaginary scene which pleases us, or a range of magnificent colours such as gold, silver, green, indigo or violet, calming peaceful colours which will aid our meditation). We should then just sit still with slow gentle thoughts passing in and out of our minds freely flowing without any emotion attached to them, regardless of any emotion such thoughts would normally attract, all the time being aware of our breathing; breathing slowly in and out, calmly and peacefully. The time spend doing this meditation may vary considerably depending upon how much time we can spare and in some cases he importance of a session in respect to our stress loading at any given period.

MASSAGE

In terms of physical stress relief methods, massage can certainly prove to be one of the most effective. Whether it is carried out by a partner, friend, or professional therapist, in terms of physical relaxation, the benefits of such a treatment are quite indisputable. There are however certain rules which apply if such a therapy is to be undertaken, particularly where unskilled persons are carrying out the massage.

First and foremost, the timing and atmosphere in respect to such treatments is very important if they are to be effective. It is no good having a relaxing massage if you have to dash off somewhere for an appointment straight afterwards, or have to deal with some stressful situations.

Ideally massage is best carried out at the end of the day, or at weekends, in a relaxing environment where you have no pressures to undo the good which such an experience can do you. Indeed part of the benefit of such treatment lies in the time allocation which you set yourself for such treatment.

Having found a suitable time to have your treatment; you then have to see that the local environment is conducive to the treatment. You need to ensure that the room is warm enough, also that the room lighting is soft (best done by using a side light rather than a central one for example). For added effect you can of course use candlelight and your favourite soft music. It's also important to make sure the phone is disconnected, and that if you have any children, that they are either out; or in bed, all can make a considerable difference to the quality of your massage. The main drawback with massage however, is that we need someone else to do it for us and sadly, not everyone is skilled in respect to carrying out such a treatment.

When carrying out a treatment much will depend upon how well you know the person you're giving the treatment to, as to where and when you work on them. In all cases the task will be very strenuous; and so you will need to be appropriately dressed for the occasion. (It's important to wear a short-sleeved top for example, so that you don't brush against the skin of the person you're giving a massage to). It's also important to ensure that your nails are fairly short and can't scratch the person having the massage (you should also remove any hand jewellery for the same reason).

Before starting the massage, it's important to ensure that the person having the massage is comfortable, and that they have removed as much of their jewellery as possible i.e. watches, rings, necklaces, bracelets etc. It is also essential to ensure that your hands (and any oil you might use) are warm before you start, and to ensure that the person having the massage is kept warm. Where necessary, the person should be covered with linen towels; with each working area only exposed when you are working on that particular region (though this does very much depend upon the room temperature, and patient's preference of course).

For anyone who is not used to giving massages to others, its important to realise just how tiring giving such treatments to others can be, and just how much energy a masseur will use during a massage. It is also important to be aware of your posture when giving a massage too, as bad posture can lead to the masseur having painful hip or back problems if their subject is not positioned correctly. Ideally a person should be lying on a proper massage table so that they are fairly high up and so the masseur does not have to lean over them too much or stretch. It is also important that the masseur has all round access to the person being treated and can walk round them to treat all areas.

Sadly not everyone has access to a massage table and so many massages are carried out on a bed, which although not ideal, can still provide a suitable massage area to work as far as the person having the treatment is concerned. Ideally the bed will need to have a firm mattress with possibly a sheet of plywood to stop the bed surface from being too spongy, so that the masseur can carry out firm movements against a solid base. Probably the greatest disadvantage to working on a bed however, lies in respect to the person giving the massage. With such a low the working height, the masseur will be forced to bend over the person having the massage, which could cause back and pain injuries if not carried out efficiently.

As will all physical activities, it is important to keep your back as straight as possible whilst working on someone. This means working at a reasonable distance from the person being massaged, so that you are leaning into your subject at an angle, keeping your back as straight as possible, rather than being stooped over them or twisting your back and hips at close quarters in a cramped manner. It's best to stand alongside your subject starting at their ankle working up the legs in long straight strokes. Where working areas are cramped, this is particularly bad for the masseur. In some instances where the upper body only needs treatment, it might be better to get the person having the treatment to sit in a chair (preferably a narrow, straight backed chair with no padded wings so as to allow easy access for the masseur). You can then comfortably massage their neck and shoulders without any impediments.

As regards the massage movements, whilst there are many intricate movements that can be carried out during a massage, the basic movements involve the fingertips, the flat of the hand, the heel of the hand, the thumbs; or the thumbs and first fingers together.

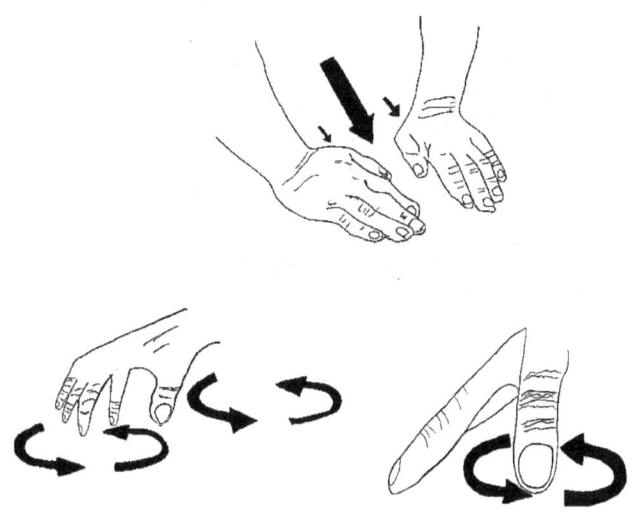

To start off with opening strokes called effleurage are used, whereby the flat of the hand will be used, following the contours of the area being worked on i.e. the legs, arms or back, pushing upwards with the fingers and the flat of the hand and then back downward repeating this movement several times, to warm up the body tissue being worked on (usually using both hands side by side with the fingertips closed and angled slightly towards each other). Once the surface tissue is relaxed, then deeper muscular movements tend to follow. Firstly the fingertips may be used in circular motions (i.e. finger frictions) or in some parts of the body the thumbs will be used in circular motions (i.e. thumb frictions on the hands for example)

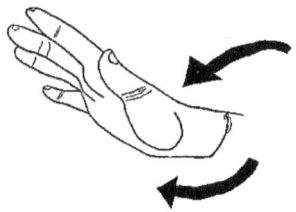

then particularly on the legs, the heel on the hand will be used, pushing firmly up the leg with thumb frictions being used as appropriate afterwards.

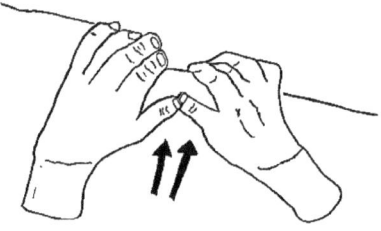

On the back of the leg, thigh, hips and shoulders, a movement called pettrisage will also be used; this involves rolling the larger muscles backwards and forwards between your thumb and first finger. With the hands and the soles of the feet crossover movements will be made with the thumbs.

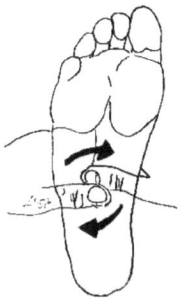

On the feet for example the masseur will place the underside of their fingers on the persons' foot, then using both their thumbs (end to end) to grip the sole of the foot at the base of the ankle; they will then effleurage the foot by sliding their hands up the foot pulling off the toes and starting all over again, doing this several times. The masseur will then massage the foot, by sliding their thumbs backward and forwards, sliding gradually along the sole of the foot being treated towards the toes. As a form of stress relief, this procedure (a mini foot massage can be a most effective treatment in its own right when someone has been on their feet all day).

There are other movements that can be used such as tapotement where the fingers are tapped/vibrated in sequence very quickly, usually on bony areas where too much pressure would be harmful or uncomfortable, (areas such as the chest-bone for example). This movement can also be applied to areas of the face too; for facial massage movements have to be very gentle and flowing for obvious reasons. In several of these manoeuvres, the first two forefingers are lined up end to end along certain areas (i.e. the lips and eyebrows), then pulled apart slowly and firmly; this is done several times as part of the mouth muscle treatment. With these areas a second movement involves

In respect to the order and areas worked on - it is pretty much up to the person giving the massage as to whether to start on the front or the back, both are acceptable. The most important thing to remember is that you must work equally on both sides of the person having the massage, i.e. both arms and legs. Failure to do so will give the person a strange sensation of feeling lopsided. It is also essential for medical reasons that you always work towards the heart.

For practical reasons it is often a good policy to start with the person having the massage lying on their back, since they will inevitably relax more and more as the treatment progresses (even to the point of drifting off to sleep in some cases). This being the case, it is important to get those areas done first where you are likely to require their co-operation, i.e. the arms, and in respect to the moving of any pillows; so that you can work on their neck in an effective way.

In respect to the massage strokes themselves, they are not as intricate as they might appear to the untrained eye. In actual fact there are about six basic strokes involved. All use either the flat of the hand, the heel of the hand, the fingertips, the thumbs, or all together.

As I've already indicated, sometimes the moves are of a stroking nature, at other times, a kneading, tapping, or a circular motion will be employed (depending upon the area you are working on, and the stage you are at within that area).

In respect to the pressures used; much will depend upon the instructions coming from the person having the treatment, and their particular body frame. In order to prevent your massage movements dragging and causing possible friction burns; it is important to use a massage medium of some kind. This may be a vegetable oil of some type, or alternative talcum powder, depending upon your own preference, or the person's having the treatment.

Since the following movements vary greatly depending upon whether you are working on the front or back, I will for the purposes of clarity, give the following directions in respect to the patient lying on their back, and then cover any variations of movement on the reverse side later.

The front of the legs

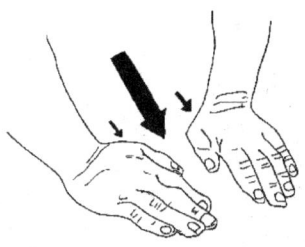

To start off you use an effleurage (or opening stroke) and generally start on the legs. Firstly you position both hands side by side at the patients' ankle, then clasping the leg firmly, push up to the top of the thigh, before coming back down again (being careful to cover the whole lower leg), with both hands moving beside each other in total harmony. This has the effect of both warming up the area; and most importantly, relaxing the body tissue, ready for the more vigorous movements which follow. (This opening stroke is the same, no matter whether you are working on a person's front or back.)

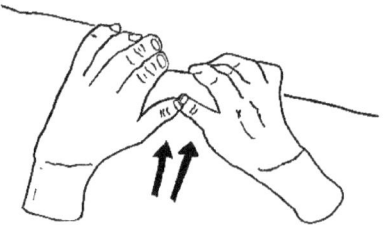

Once the body tissue feels warm and soft (generally after half a dozen or so passes over the leg). You can then start on the deeper friction (petrisage) movements, starting with the lower leg; though whether or not you do these, will very much depend upon your level of confidence; and the time available to you of course.

Having loosened up the lower leg, you then need to work in a circular motion with your thumbs up the outside edge of the leg bone, from the ankle, up to the knee-cap. Having done this several times, you may then move to the bulky muscles at the side of the main leg bone.

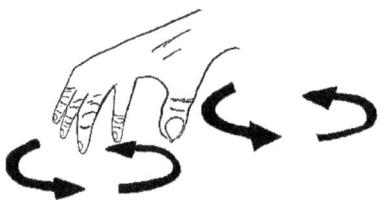

To work on these, you use the fingertips, again in a circular motions (called finger frictions), up to the knee and back down the leg to the ankle several times. Having completed this movement, you are then able to move on to the kneecap itself, though this will depend upon the sensitivity of the person having the treatment (as some people dislike having their kneecaps touched). If you do decide to work on the kneecap, you do so by using your fingertips and thumb, working carefully round the joint in a circular motion. Once you have completed this movement, you can then move on to the thigh. Again you should start of with an effleurage stroke, pushing firmly with the flat of both your hands up towards the groin. You should then return slowly back down to the knee, being sure to cover the whole of the thigh, fanning out your hands as much as you can.

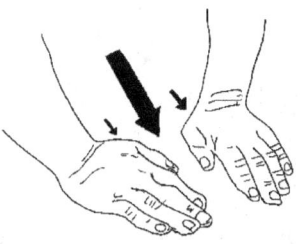

Having carried out this effleurage stroke half a dozen times or so, you can then start on some deeper movements. To perform these, you need to stand parallel to the person's thigh and physically knead the tissue between your fingertips, being careful to do so in a firm but careful way. You should then slide one hand forward and one hand backward right round the thigh as far and as much as you can, working in lines; right up to the top of the thigh, gripping the loose flesh between your fingers and thumbs. Having completed this movement several times, you can then slide down to the person's foot and do some effleurage strokes on the foot itself (provided the patient has no objections). These can be done by carefully gripping the contours of the foot between your hands, one above and one underneath, with the top one doing circular motions. You can then do some gentle kneading motions on the top of the foot with your thumbs, covering the whole top surface of the foot and pushing round the ankles towards the toes and up the calf of the leg.

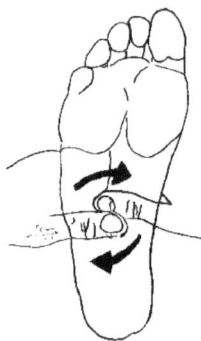

To massage the soles of the feet you need to interlock both hands on the top surface of the persons' feet. You should then cross your thumbs together beneath the patient's feet and pull them apart, backwards and forwards in a sawing motion, whilst at the same time, sliding up and down the foot, before finally taking your hands off their feet at the persons' toes and then repeat this manoeuvre several times working from the persons' ankle towards their toes. Once you have completed these manoeuvres, you should then do a closing stroke covering the whole leg in the same way that you did when you started, by pushing up the leg with the flat or your hand, following up the contours of the leg with your fingertips. Once you have completed this manoeuvre half a dozen times or so, you can then go on to repeat the same moves on the other leg.

     Ideally the legs should take around ten minutes to do (roughly five minutes a leg), though this does vary according to how quick you work the area. Having completed the legs, you are then free to do the stomach, though again this is optional, since not everyone likes having their stomach massaged.

The stomach

In order to do the stomach you need to position your hands very carefully; since there is little room for manoeuvre with this part of our anatomy.

First of all you should line up your hands at diagonal angles, with your thumbs outstretched; so that the gap between them and your fingertips becomes a diamond. Once you have this shape you are then able to carry out the effleurage (opening stroke).

With your thumbs lined up just above the patients' waste-band and your fingertips on the patients' navel you slowly push upwards, then when your fingertips reach the patient's ribcage; you pull both hands outwards away from each other, following the line of the lowest rib. When you reach waistband level; you should then bring your hands together again and repeat the same process several times. Having carried out this manoeuvre, you should then (with your right or left hand) place your chosen hand to the left of the patient's navel and rub round it in a circular clockwise motion; as far as you can. Having done so, you should then follow on closely behind with your other hand, so that you complete a circle, again you complete this motion several times (always in a clockwise fashion).

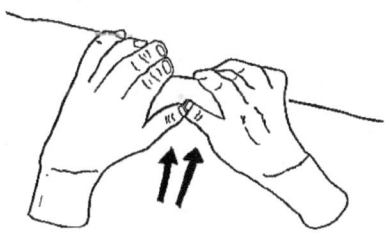

Having completed this manoeuvre, you should then move round beside the persons' stomach. Using your fingertips and thumbs, you should then knead the loose flesh at the persons' sides, between the persons' ribs and hips (as you did on the persons' thighs), working both towards the ribs and the pelvis alternately on both sides. Once both sides are thoroughly kneaded, you should then finish off by repeating the diamond stroke that you started with. The stomach itself should take around 5 minutes to do. Next come the arms, which should take around 7 minutes to do.

The arms

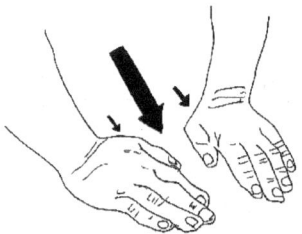

Starting with the forearm, you should work upwards from the wrist using the same effleurage (stroking) moves as you did on the lower leg, but being careful to support the persons' arm as you work on it.

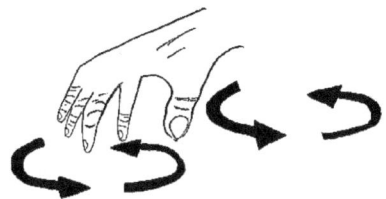

    Once you have warmed up the arm and done enough finger frictions (rotating finger circles up the arm), you can then move on up to do the upper arm in the same way that you did the patient's thigh, being careful to support the patient's arm as you do so.
    Having completed the arm itself, you are then able to move back down to do the hands. To do them you should first perform an opening stroke by running your hand diagonally across the patients' palm, locking your thumb with their thumb and pulling yours down from theirs; you should then repeat the process several times.

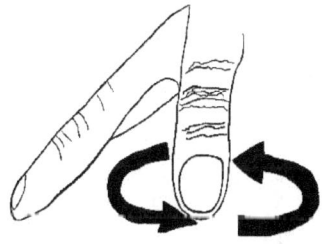

Once you have completed this manoeuvre you should then do some circular thumb frictions around the bases of the thumb and the palm of the hand. You should then turn the hand over and do some circular thumb frictions over the back of the hand.

Once you have covered the back of the hand, you should then grip the top of each of your patient's finger firmly (but not too tightly), between your thumb and first finger. You should then slowly pull your thumb and finger downwards, rotating them as you go, repeating the process several times on each finger. Finally you should repeat the diagonal opening stroke across the palm of the hand, pulling downwards off of the thumb.

Once you have completed this finishing stroke on the first hand you should then move round to the other side of the person. You should then repeat the whole process, starting again with the upper and lower arm, working in the same way that you massaged the patient's leg, being sure to support their arm.

Once you have completed the arms, you should then move round to the back of the person's head. Having positioned yourself comfortably behind the person, you should then pull the cushion on which their head is resting, slightly backwards so that you can get your hands under their neck and shoulders, at the same time making sure that they are comfortable.

The upper torso

Once you are sure your patient is comfortable, you can then start to work on their chest, shoulders and neck all in one go. The movements involved in this manoeuvre will depend upon whether you are working on a man or woman (and in the case of women, how well you know them). When working on women, it's necessary for them to unclip their bra and slide out of the straps as well, to give you access to their shoulders. In order to preserve their modesty it is therefore wise to cover their chest with a towel beforehand, so as to spare them any embarrassment.

(Full) male upper torso

If you are working on a man then their whole chest will more than likely be exposed before you and you can be much freer with your movements, using much bigger strokes. Being a large working area; it's important to ensure that you have enough of the chosen massage medium on the patient before you start working on them. By doing so there is far less risk of causing friction burns on the persons' neck (which is likely to get very sore after a while if there is insufficient lubrication whilst carrying out such movements).

Initially when new to doing this manoeuvre, it is best to place a reservoir of oil or talk just below the shoulders on each side, so that you can top up your hand coverage should your hands run dry through insufficient application. This is particularly applicable where a man has a very hairy chest in order to prevent hair drag, which can be very painful for the person having the treatment.

When you are ready to start the massage itself, you should place both hands firmly on the top of the shoulders, with the fingertips pointing slightly inward. You should then move towards the ribs using the flat of the hand, working in a figure of eight movement, back up to the neck (to the base of the spine), being sure to fan out your hands as appropriate, so as to cover the whole of the man's chest. Carefully fanning your hands out beneath the patient's shoulders, doing circular motions with your fingertips; before starting the procedure over and over again, for at least half a dozen times.

Once you have completed these opening strokes, you are then free to start some circular knuckle frictions; as you have previously done with your fingers and thumbs, on the persons' sternum (breastbone). (When carrying out this manoeuvre it's important not to apply too much pressure).

Having completed this manoeuvre, you can then continue with firm finger frictions, across the rest of the person's chest. Once you have done a series of these movements, you can then do some kneading movements in a circular motion, both up the back of the neck, and also, on the top of the shoulders and behind them as well with your fingertips. Finally you should finish off with some long strokes covering the whole chest, neck, and shoulders, just as you did when you started. In all the manoeuvres should take between 5 – 7 minutes to perform.

(Selective) Female Upper Torso

When working on women you have to work slightly differently of course, in many cases the range of movements will be greatly limited in respect to the chest region for obvious anatomical reasons. If however you know the person you are working on very well then you do indeed have a much greater scope in respect to the movements used. As a general rule however, in most cases you will merely massage round the neck and shoulders, working towards the sternum (breastbone) and back again, up the back of the neck to the base of the skull. You should then repeat the movement as you would on a man; using knuckle frictions over the sternum. You should then go straight to the shoulders and back of the neck using firm finger frictions, in a circular motion. Finally you should finish off with some longer effleurage strokes (completing a circuit) as you did when you started, working round the shoulders to the sternum (breastbone) and then back up to the base of the skull.

(Full) Female Upper Torso

Where you know a female patient well however, you can adapt your movements so that they more resemble the way you would normally massage a man, though she would of course need to be topless for you to do so.
    When undertaking this option, you start off in the normal way, working from the shoulders. When you reach the top of the breasts however, instead of pulling back to the neck, you should pick up your hands and rotate them on your fingertips (whilst still maintaining contact). You should then flip your fingers over, so that the back of your fingers are lined up together, flat between the breasts, where the working area is narrowed.

Gradually; as you have more working space, you can then fan out your hands so that they are pressed firmly on the rest of the ribcage, below the breasts. You should then pull them back towards you (whilst still maintaining contact), up the outside edge of the ribs and breast, up to the armpit and back round the shoulders again as your opening effleurage stroke.

With the top layer of underwear removed you can then continue with knuckle frictions from the neck, down between the breasts, and back up again, before continuing on to do the neck and shoulders specifically. As a final manoeuvre, you should then repeat the moves as I've just described.

Whilst such movements may at first appear to infringe upon the modesty of the person undergoing the treatment, they are in fact most beneficial for several reasons. Firstly, they allow continuity of movement across the upper torso, secondly and most importantly, these movements allow the masseur to work fully on the sternum (the main crossover point for lymphatic fluids into the bloodstream).

The suggested movements also allow the masseur to move and stimulate the lymphatics, across the whole upper body; to and from the main lymph nodes under the arm, and to the sternum (breastbone). This being the case, such movements can prove invaluable in respect to clearing away any toxins which have been disturbed during the massage; hence their inclusion in this book.

Having completed the upper torso, you then have to decide whether to do a facial massage or go straight on to do the person's other side.

Head/facial massage

As I've just indicated, it can be extremely beneficial to cover as much of the body as possible, and so it is advisable where time allows, to do some sort of facial treatment, though not necessarily an in depth one.

Massaging the face is probably the hardest part of the body to work on, in that there are so many different contours involved, and no large surface areas to work on. This being the case, a complex set of manoeuvres is required to carry out a treatment comfortably.

To carry out facial massage successfully, it is necessary to carry out the same manoeuvres as I've just described for the full female torso, i.e. using the back sides of the fingers and fingertips themselves.

The opening effleurage (stroking) strokes are carried out with the flattened fingertips working from the neck up, over the chin, up the cheeks, and round the forehead. You should then work back down the face to the neck again (a process which like other sets of opening strokes; should be carried out at least a half a dozen times or more).

Having done all the opening strokes, you should then place the backs of your fingertips on the patient's forehead, side by side; and gently push them apart in the direction of each temple. When you have done so several times, you should then select an eyebrow to work on.

To massage the eyebrows, you should place your second finger outstretched on the outer edge of the selected eyebrow and draw it up the eyebrow; closely following on a bit farther along the eyebrow with the second finger from your other hand. You should repeat these steps until you have been over the whole eyebrow several times; you should then do the other eyebrow accordingly.

Having finished the eyebrows, you should then start work on the eye sockets themselves though this is an extremely delicate task to carry out, and so those with a clumsy disposition may be better off bypassing this particular manoeuvre.

To massage the eye socket; you should start off with the back side of your second fingertip (i.e. the nail side), resting alongside the bridge of the nose, at the corner of the patient's eye. You should then, slowly and carefully; draw your fingertips along the upper contour of the sockets, towards the patients' temple, pausing when you reach the outer edge of the patient's eye socket. After a short interval you should slowly move along the lower edge of the eye socket; towards your starting point at the bridge of the nose.

When you have carried out this manoeuvre several times (very carefully); you should then massage the nose using one fingertip on each side, in circular motions, before moving outwards to do the same motion on the cheeks; but this time using all fingertips.

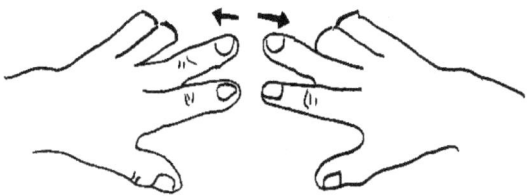

Having massaged the cheeks sufficiently; you should then move on to do the patient's lips. In order to carry out this manoeuvre you need to use both second and third fingers, placing both second fingertips end to end across the upper lips, and both third fingers upon the lower ones. Once your fingers are in place; you should then slowly draw them apart firmly along the lip, first one side then the other, repeating the process several times.

Once you have completed all these complex manoeuvres; you should then move down to the neck and repeat the very first effleurage movements that you started with, finishing off at the patient's forehead.

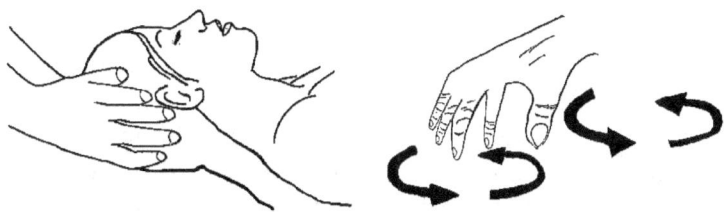

Provided your hands are not too oily; you can then start to massage the person's scalp, by spreading out your fingers and working round the head and scalp in circular motions.

Having carried out this last manoeuvre, you then have to get the person having the massage to get up and turn over onto their stomach so that you can do their back and legs. In all the manoeuvres should take between 5 – 7 minutes to carry out.

Before you can start on the persons' back, you first need to ensure that the person having the massage is comfortable and can breathe. Much will depend upon the surface you are working on as to how this may be achieved, but in all cases it is important to ensure that the person's neck is straight, with their chin and forehead well supported.

The back of the legs

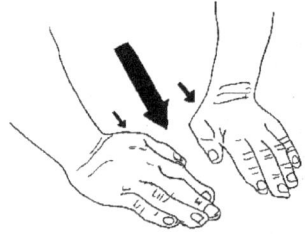

To do the back of the legs you should start with long slow effleurage strokes, using the flat of the hand in long continual strokes, from the ankle, right up to the thigh and back down again. You should repeat this process several times, being sure to cover the whole of the leg.

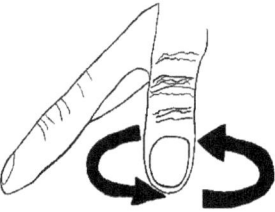

Once the leg is sufficiently warm, you can then start some gentle thumb frictions (circular movements with the thumbs) on the lower part of the leg, working up and down the leg in lines.

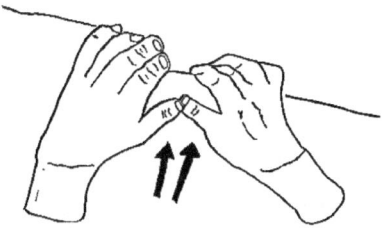

You should then move along the selected leg, rolling the muscle from side to side using your fingers and thumb, working backwards and forwards along the full length of the muscle.

Having carried out these manoeuvres, you can then repeat these moves on the upper thigh, though in most cases this will require a good deal more effort and a much firmer grip. Once you have covered the whole leg, you then finish off with those long effleurage strokes from the ankle right up to the thigh, using the flat of the hand; being sure to cover the whole of the leg's surface. Having done so, you should repeat all these manoeuvres on the other leg. In all the back of the legs should take between 5 – 7 minutes to do.

Once the legs have been fully massaged, it is then time to start on the back, which for most people is by far the most satisfying part of a massage treatment and should take around 20 minutes to do.

The buttocks/back

From the masseur's point of view, the back is probably the most exhausting area to work on, in that it is an extremely large surface area with, much stretching and reaching involved. For best effect, the back is generally worked on from all four sides, starting from the lower back upwards, then from either the left or right side, followed by the head end, working towards the buttocks, then finally from the last remaining side.

In respect to the massaging of the back itself, it is largely down to individual choice as to whether or not to include the buttocks, but in the main it is recommended that they are included. (Being a major bank of muscles, they are just as likely to harbour various harmful chemical waste products of one sort or another.) It is also more conducive to the effect of the massage to include them; by doing so you are able to cover the whole of the person's posterior side from head to toe.

Having decided to do the buttocks, you should then pull down any obscuring undergarments so that they are exposed, and then include the buttocks as a part of the back.

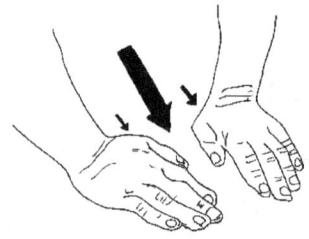

Having lubricated your hands thoroughly, you should then place your hands flat at the base of the person's spine, just above the buttocks, and slowly push upwards in a figure of eight movement; up to, and round the shoulders. You should then move back down to your starting position, and up over the buttocks themselves in a smaller figure of eight, before returning to the centre of the spine to start these movements all over again. Once the body tissue is sufficiently warmed up and relaxed, you can then concentrate on more specialised movements.

After positioning yourself alongside the person you are giving the massage to, you should then start kneading each buttock individually, occasionally fanning outwards with the flat of your hand, gripping the tissue between your thumb and first finger and pushing up towards the hip. After you have carried out these moves, you can then concentrate upon the back itself. It's generally best to start off with some gentle stretching manoeuvres with the flat of the hand as you have done previously. You should then cross your thumbs back and forwards at the base of the spine (one immediately above the other).

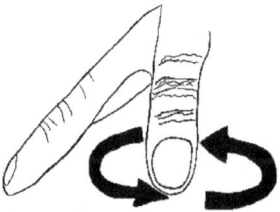

Following the line of the pelvic girdle, you should then gradually work outwards, using circular motions with the thumbs, doing this several times out towards the hip and back towards the spine again.

You should then align your two thumbs either side of the spine and gently work in circular movements from the top of the buttocks, up the spine, towards the base of the skull, before coming back down and starting again. You should finish off by working around the shoulders in a figure of eight, before finally coming back down to your starting position, maintaining physical contact all the way.

When you feel you have done enough work on this shoulder tissue, you should then turn your attention to the larger muscles on the outer edges of the back, working up, down, and from side to side, across the person's back.

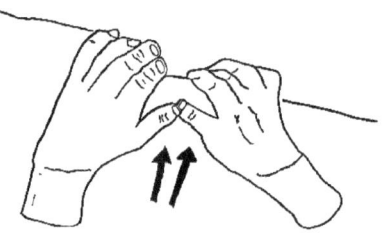

    Having worked thoroughly on the main back muscles, you should then turn your attention to the shoulders again, carefully kneading them between your thumb and fingertips, continuing up to the base of the skull. You should then come back down to the shoulders again before repeating these movements all over again, followed by some firm effleurage (stroking) type movements in a figure of eight towards the neck.

    Having satisfied yourself that the neck and shoulder muscles are sufficiently relaxed, you should then work on each shoulder blade, and the bordering cavities; working carefully with your thumb, round the edges of each shoulder-blade in circular motions. You should then work on the muscle covering the shoulder-blade itself with your fingers; again in circular motions.

    Once the shoulders have been sufficiently worked on, you should then move round so that you are positioned behind the persons' head and start again, working on their whole back.

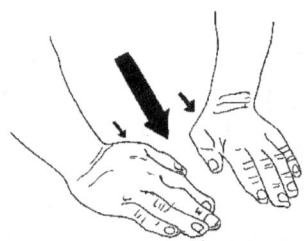

Just as you did before, you should star off with some basic effleurage strokes; working from the shoulders, down to the buttocks in a figure of eight, in the same way that you did the back from the other end, when you started.

When you have done half a dozen or so effleurage strokes, you should then do some stretching exercises, starting with one hand at the base on the patient's spine, and the other at the shoulder. Pressing down firmly with each hand, you should then push them in opposite directions, so that they meet in the middle of the back, reversing these manoeuvres as appropriate.

Having completed these manoeuvres, you should then work with the heel of each hand in circular motions up and down the spine several times, making sure that your hands are well lubricated, so as not to cause any friction burns to your patient. You should then finish off with some finger frictions, before moving up to work again on the neck and shoulders.

When working on the neck and shoulders, you should use both your fingertips and thumbs, working in circular motions, both up the neck and along each shoulder in turn, also doing the tops of the arms as well with the ball of the hand. Finally you should do a series of effleurage strokes covering the whole back as you did when you started, pushing firmly up and down the muscles of the patients' back.

Whilst maintaining contact with the person having the massage, you should then move round to work on them from the last side, positioning yourself by their hip. You should then repeat all the moves you did on their other side, starting off with effleurage (stroking movements), over the whole back (including the buttocks, where appropriate). You should then work on those specific areas as you did before, i.e. the buttocks, central spine, bordering muscles, shoulders and neck.

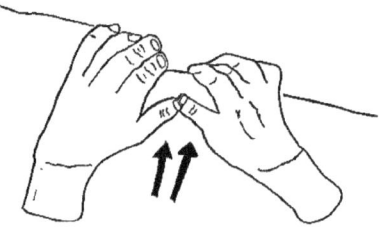

To do the buttocks, you should again knead and roll them between your fingers and thumbs, working on each one in turn. You should then cross your thumbs backwards and forwards at the base of the spine, gradually working outwards, following the line of the pelvic girdle, using circular motions with the thumbs. You should do this several times, backwards and forwards, before continuing these circular movements up and down either side of the spine.

You should then work on those outer back muscles which you did earlier on, both from side to side and across the back; working up to the shoulders and back down to the buttocks again.

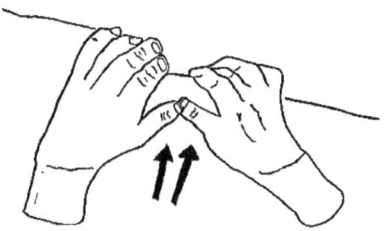

You should then work on the neck and shoulders, kneading them between your fingers and thumbs in the same way that you did before. You should then work in circular motions around the edge of the shoulder blade using your thumbs, before doing some finger frictions in circular motions on the top of the shoulder blade, followed by some firm effleurage type movements in a figure of eight towards the neck.

When these moves have been done, you should then finish off with some final effleurage strokes covering the whole of the back and buttocks, in the same way that you did when you started on the person.

Finally you should cover the person's back again to keep them warm, then leave them to rest for a while.

AROMATHERAPY HOME TREATMENTS

As a home treatment, aromatherapy has become extremely popular during the past few years, due to considerable publicity from women's magazines, national newspaper columns, and a wealth of training courses run by local practitioners.

Besides being used to enhance conventional massage treatment, aromatherapy/essential oils have a very wide range of uses, and can influence a great many conditions in a positive way. It is important to realise however, that these essences are in effect medicines and should therefore be treated as such. Sadly many of them are sold over the counter and through mail order with little or no instruction as to their use.

Oil production methods

Aromatherapy oils can vary tremendously in cost and quality, depending upon their source and type of manufacture, jasmin being a prime example. There are two main sources of this essence, both of differing quality, which does of course reflect in their price.

Mediterranean jasmin for example costs twice the price of Egyptian jasmin, thus reflecting its superior quality. In buying the lower priced oils you also run the risk of purchasing products which have no therapeutic benefits whatsoever.

As regards the authentic essences themselves, they are produced through a variety of ways, though there are basically four recognised techniques used for their extraction.

The first method is of course crushing, or expression as it is technically called. This is by far the simplest form of extraction. This method is often used to remove fluids from citrus fruits. The oil is physically squeezed from the rind of the relevant fruit, and is by far the cheapest of processes.

Another way of removing oils is through solvent extraction. This method is used to extract resins and gums from tree bark. Also some flowers are treated in this way. The materials are placed in a vat, usually of acetone and boiled. During this process, the solvent concerned absorbs the oil and is then processed further by using alcohol to separate out the valuable oil from the surrounding debris.

The third method of extraction, is a much simpler process, that of distillation, whereby the oils are steamed out (usually from the leaves of plants). The oils are then skimmed off and processed yet further, to ensure their purity.

Finally we have a process called enfleurage, where the oils are extracted from the flowers themselves. This is an extremely costly and time consuming process, since many millions of blooms are needed to produce a small amount of oil, hence the astronomical cost of these oils. This process applies particularly to rose oil, jasmine, and orange blossom (or neroli as it is more commonly known).

Basically the flowers are placed upon a layer of fat and left for the juices to be absorbed into it. For some, this fat will need to be hot to work properly. For others cold fat is quite sufficient. When the fat has been completely saturated, it is dissolved in alcohol, and the oils are then processed and blended.

These processes may sound rather severe for such sensitive material, but surprising as it may seem; they have no effect upon the oil's potency whatsoever. In fact the oils are more likely to be damaged through bad storage than anything else, as I shall explain later.

Their versatility

The plant extracts themselves are in effect vegetable hormones; and have been designed by mother-nature to withstand a wide variety of chemicals and natural acids. (This also applies when they enter our bodies during an aromatherapy massage for example.) Direct massage absorption is only one of many ways in which these oils can be used. They can also for example, be used for therapeutic effect at bath-time, by simply adding a few drops of oil to your bathwater. To be most effective in this respect, the oils should be mixed with an aromatherapy milk of some kind, otherwise, being oil based, they will not mix with the waters of your bath.

Essential oils can also be used as inhalations (taken up through the nasal passages to relieve a cold by way of steam). A modern favourite among these oils is eucalyptus, though most oils of herbal and spicy type, i.e. camphor, cinnamon, cloves and ginger etc, can have great effect when used in this way. Many of these oils can shorten a cold's effects drastically and bring about great relief at night, particularly when a few drops of these oils are put on a handkerchief or a pillowcase. When used in this way, it's very important to realise that these oils will sting if they come into contact with sensitive areas of our bodies; they should not therefore be allowed to come into contact with the eyes. When using these types of oil for inhalation relief, the eyes should therefore be kept closed until the vapour has dispersed. The same applies in the case of commercial brand; off the shelf inhalation products as well of course, in that they use the same types of oils in their preparations.

As well as for infusions, aromatherapy oils can also be added to face creams and shampoos, provided the person blending them has had a degree of training, or has read up thoroughly on the subject. Ideally the base waxes and carrier oils used should be free of artificial chemicals and preferably unscented. Once you have found such mediums, you can then add a few drops of an appropriate essential oil. Camomile, for example, is sometimes added to shampoo, and is known to be good for the hair and scalp. In the case of facial massage, a wide variety of oils are suitable, depending upon a person's requirements.

Once again a suitable carrier medium will be needed, preferably almond or hazelnut oil of cosmetic quality. As for the essential oils themselves, lavender is particularly good for oily and spotty skins, where infection is prevalent. As a tonic, jasmin or neroli would probably be a better choice, since they are known to improve the elasticity of the skin and are often used in face creams.

Of course the most important thing to remember when using these ingredients is that the blend must first be warmed up, so as to improve its absorption through the porous network of the skin, so that it can do its job. Once such oils are absorbed into the body, they can carry out an almost infinite amount of tasks. They can even be used very effectively to treat foot disorders such as athlete's foot and verucas for example; by simply rubbing a few drops of tea tree oil into the affected areas you can often relieve such conditions.

For anyone still uncertain about using essential oils, they would be well advised to consult their nearest therapist or pharmacist, since many health food shops and high street chemists do stock such things as herbal shampoos and face creams of the type I have just mentioned.

Safety considerations

Where aromatherapy oils are purchased over the counter, and through mail order in undiluted form, it s wise to be wary of them; they should never be regarded as a wholly safe cure all. You will probably realise from what I said earlier, much will depend upon how they have been produced; this being so, their purity cannot always be guaranteed.

Whilst some oils such as tea tree and peppermint can be used to treat conditions such as mouth ulcers, toothache, sore gums, digestive disorders etc they should never be taken internally via the mouth, or drunk in suspension, without the supervision of a qualified therapist or doctor. When you are buying oils, always be wary of low priced ones as their cost often reflects their quality.

As regards their storage and what to look out for - the main things to note when purchasing the oils, as well as their price, is how they have been stored. Whilst they are quite resistant to many chemicals, they are like most things, susceptible to sunlight, which will destroy their potency very quickly. They should always be kept in dark glass bottles (either green, brown or blue) and of course should always be clearly labelled.

Never buy essential oils (or store them) in clear glass, for the reason I have just mentioned. Also never buy or store essential oils in plastic bottles since they are prone to leaching i.e. absorbing the plastics that surround them.

You may well know from what I said earlier, that many of the oils have been washed or extracted using some kind of alcohol or solvent. If you think about it, plastic will literally melt when it comes into contact with solvents. Sadly and this is exactly what will happen in the case of the bottles; not necessarily so that the bottle will leak, but certainly enough for the oil to absorb some of the plastic's chemicals, which if taken internally could be carcinogenic, or damage the liver.

Respect the oils for what they are, in that they are bottled in a concentrated form, and could if misused, be dangerous. Many of the oils including citrus and peppermint can cause rashes and allergic reactions if applied directly onto sensitive skins; that's why professional therapists often carry out a patch test before carrying out a full treatment using such oils.

There are some oils, particularly bergamot, which are photo-sensitive and therefore could present a health risk if the user applied them before going out to sunbathe or before lying on a sun-bed. Their various strengths could also be a problem in that some are applied at one per cent strength, whilst others can be as much as five per cent. Few of the suppliers currently give such details, or any other warnings come to that. A great many oils are unsuitable for use during pregnancy too (oils such as rosemary, peppermint and juniper being typical examples).

Fortunately a great many books have been written on the subject of aromatherapy in recent years, all of which give details as to what the various oils can do. Whilst such books can be very informative, it's essential that people read them thoroughly, and note any warnings that are given by the author.

Oils such as cypress and juniper for example, are often stated as fluid reducing agents (or diuretics as they are professionally known). In the wrong concentration, or used without supervision, these oils could cause serious damage to a person's kidneys or liver. Whilst I have no wish to undermine people's confidence in these oils, it is important to realise this when using them for the first time. In the right hands, when used by well qualified and knowledgeable person, they are both a safe and a wholly effective alternative to the various drug related therapies currently at our disposal. As I have already indicated however, they are in effect medicines, and should therefore be treated as such.

CLOSING STATEMENT

Whilst it is hoped that the information in this guide has proved helpful, it is important to note however, that the methods of treatment in this guide are often subject to subtle variation depending upon the therapist undertaking a particular treatment. In the case of massage for example, few masseurs follow the exact same treatment order or carry out exactly the same movements. Likewise with aromatherapy treatments; the oils used are subject to regular review in respect to both their efficacy and also their long-term safety. The same applies greatly to dietary advice and regimes too.

Whilst a particular food or diet may be highly recommended by one particular body of experts at one point, it may be the case that another body of experts carrying out research, draw completely different conclusions in respect to a particular food's efficacy in respect to staving off certain types of illness; with the reverse being true in some cases. This has happened in respect to health scares regarding dairy produce, i.e. full cream milk, butter verses margarine, eggs nutritional supplements etcetera. The same applies to wine and plain chocolate. Some see such products as detrimental to health, whilst others suggest they may be beneficial if consumed in moderation.

As with all advice and guidance (particularly in respect to therapies), it cannot be stressed strongly enough that it is important to have good background knowledge in respect to any therapies/treatments or diet plans before undertaking any of them, which can involve a lot of research to find both the most effective, and the safest option, which is right for you. Unfortunately due to page constraints, this guide gives only brief outline views of each therapy, and so it is up to all readers of this guide to seek out further in depth information and use the most up to date research via the internet etc when seriously considering one of the therapy options in this book before commencing any form of therapy or specialised diet.

Sadly as indicated in the opening page of this guide; whilst summarising the main "complementary" and "alternative" therapies that are available, the author of this guide can take no responsibility in respect to any treatment outcomes. As stated it is therefore up to the reader of this guide to research their chosen treatment option thoroughly before commencing any forms of treatment, as this document serves only as a rough guide.

INDEX

	Page Number
INTRODUCTION	4
PHYSICAL THERAPIES	16
Massage therapy	16
Physiotherapy/sports therapy	19
Chiropractic treatment	21
Osteopathy	24
Alexander therapy	25
Rolfing therapy	26
Kinesiology	26
Hydrotherapy	28
Chiropody	29
Colonic irrigation	31
HERBAL/FLOWER THERAPIES	32
Homeopathy	32
Bach flower remedies	33
Aromatherapy	34
ORIENTAL PRESSURE THERAPIES	42
Acupuncture	43
Shiatsu	44
Acupressure	44
Reflexology	46

INDEX

	Page Number
SPIRITUAL THERAPIES	**54**
Spiritual healers	**54**
Reiki therapy	57
HORMONAL BALANCING THERAPIES	**58**
Music and colour therapy	58
Crystal healing therapy	59
Visualisation therapy	**60**
Yoga	**60**
COUNSELLING THERAPIES	**62**
General counselling	**62**
Stress consultants	**63**
Dieticians	**64**
RELATIONSHIP COUNSELLING THERAPIES	**65**
Relationship counselling/mediation	**65**
Sex therapists	66
PSYCHOTHERAPY	67
Behavioural therapists	67
Group therapy	67
Hypnotherapy	68
Diagnostic tools	78
Kirlian photography	78

INDEX

	Page Number
Iridology	79
Dowsing	**81**
Allergy testing	**82**
SELF HELP	**84**
Off the Shelf and Internet Products	**84**
PAIN RELIEF	**85**
HOME PHYSIOTHERAPY TREATMENT	88
Strains and sprains	88
DIET AND NUTRITION	**91**
Nutritional components	**92**
Personal circumstances	**98**
Nutritional quality	**102**
Health restrictions	**105**
Women's health	113
Dieting	115
STRESS	**118**
Stress management	**120**
Stress relief	**123**
Self belief	**125**
Social interaction	**128**
Time-pressures	**132**

INDEX

	Page Number
Financial pressures	**13**3
Transport stresses	**13**5
SELF HYPNOSIS	**13**7
MEDITATION	**14**0
MASSAGE	**14**2
AROMATHERAPY HOME TREATMENTS	**17**2

www.ingramcontent.com/pod-product-compliance
Lightning Source LLC
Chambersburg PA
CBHW071536220526
45469CB00003B/801